AA

Asthma & Bronchitis

Symptoms, causes, orthodox treatment and
how herbal medicine will help.

Other published and forthcoming titles
in the series include:

IBS & Colitis

Anxiety & Tension

Migraine & Headaches

Arthritis & Rheumatism

Menopause

For full details please send for a free copy of the latest catalogue.
See back cover for address.

Asthma & Bronchitis

Jill Wright MNIMH

HERBAL HEALTH

...lom

© Copyright 2002 Jill Wright

British Library Cataloguing in Publication Data.
A catalogue record for this book is available from the British Library.

Edited by Diana Brueton
Cover design by Shireen Nathoo Design, London
Produced for How To Books by Deer Park Productions
Designed and typeset by Shireen Nathoo Design, London
Printed and bound in Great Britain by Bell & Bain Ltd., Glasgow

Note: The material contained in this book is set out in good faith for general guidance and no liability can be accepted for loss or expense incurred as a result of relying in particular circumstances on statements made in the book. The laws and regulations are complex and liable to change, and readers should check the current position with the relevant authorities before making personal arrangements.

Herbal Health *is an imprint of*
How To Books

Contents

Preface

What makes you suspect that you have asthma or bronchitis?

- Does your chest often feels tight?
- Do you break into coughing when you run for a bus?
- Do you make a high wheezy noise when you breathe out?

You may have **asthma**. If you have consulted your doctor with a persistent cough after a common cold, or noticed that your child starts coughing when they run or exercise, you may have been given a diagnosis of asthma. You or a member of your family might have had episodes of feeling unable to breathe or have had the unnerving experience of having to go to hospital because of breathing difficulties. These **asthmatic crises** may have been precipitated by a cold or chest infection, by allergy or even an intense emotional experience. You will probably be prescribed long-term medicinal inhalants to prevent recurrence of these episodes.

Bronchitis also causes

- coughing
- a sore, tight chest
- and breathing difficulties.

You may be prescribed anti-biotics, often several courses each year as infections recur.

If you suffer from either of these complaints (many people have both) you may be looking for an alternative treatment, or hoping to reduce your use of conventional medication. Herbs have been used for chest ailments for hundreds of years and many still have much to offer in these conditions.

As a member of the National Institute of Medical Herbalists, trained in herbal pharmacology, nutrition and medical sciences, I offer clear, reliable advice on the safe use of herbal medicines which will help to relieve symptoms and improve your overall health. During ten years of retail and clinical practice I have answered questions every day on how to treat respiratory problems with herbs. In this book I have set out to answer the most frequently asked questions and to give you further information if you or your family suffer from asthma and bronchitis.

Herbal medicine is the leading alternative to conventional treatment and is still the major form of medicine in many parts of the world. There are many advantages to using herbal remedies and this book will guide you simply through the process of choosing the right one.

- Discover what herbal remedies can do to reduce inflammation and infection in the airways without unpleasant side-effects.

- Learn how to combine herbs in the correct doses to

achieve an individual prescription which will help your particular problems. A brief guide to how asthma and bronchitis develop will help you plan your own herbal prescription as well as understand your treatments and get more out of visits to doctors and consultants.

- Find out more about food as medicine and how to maintain a healthy respiratory system by eating the right foods.

The advice contained in this book is for general use only. If you have an allergy, or are taking any medication or have a medical condition which may affect your use of herbal medicine, you should seek help from a qualified health care professional such as a doctor or a medical herbalist before using herbal remedies at home.

Asthmatic crises are dangerous and can lead to death. You should seek emergency medical help if you have serious breathing difficulty or are in any doubt as to the severity of the incident.

Jill Wright

❦ 1 ❦

Understanding asthma and bronchitis

All about the respiratory system

The respiratory system consists of organs and passageways
which enable oxygen to be extracted from the air and
enter our bloodstream. This includes the nose, mouth,
throat, windpipe (trachea), bronchial tubes and lungs. In
addition narrow **Eustachian tubes** run from our throat to
our ears, and help to maintain even pressure on the
eardrum. These are readily blocked when we suffer a head
cold. All the airways are lined with a special layer of cells
which are called the **ciliary mucous membrane**. This
membrane contains cells which constantly produce thin
mucus, a starchy liquid which helps the absorption of
oxygen and traps noxious substances such as dust and
pollen. The mucus, along with entrapped irritants, is
moved upwards for expulsion via nose and mouth, by
minute hair-like cells called **cilia**, which are constantly
brushing the airways clean in a motion known as the
ciliary escalator. This may be affected by environmental
pollutants and infections, as you will find out later. In
addition to mucus and hair cells, white blood cells are to

be found along the airways and help provide immunity to infections.

The nose

Air is drawn in through the nose, which contains a series of bony 'baffles', like a series of interspaced seaside-windbreaks. These mucus covered structures humidify the air, which bounces around, depositing foreign particles. These are expelled by the ciliary hairs, and more forcefully by the sneeze reflex, which responds to intense irritation.

The windpipe and bronchial tubes

The windpipe – **trachea** – lies in front of your gullet, so you can feel its muscular shape on the outside of your throat. When you eat it is closed at the top by a flap called the **epiglottis**. If this remains a little open during eating, and food particles stray into your trachea, a fit of violent coughing will occur by reflex to clear the airway.

The trachea branches at its end into right and left **bronchi**, which further branch into smaller tubes called **bronchioles**. The trachea, bronchi and bronchioles have muscular walls which can relax causing dilation, or contract causing constriction. This is necessary for the changes in air intake due to exercise or cold weather. Normally bronchial tubes are maintained at almost maximal dilation, and are constricted in response to irritation (by bacteria, allergens or pollutants). They are also lined with ciliary mucous membrane.

Respiratory muscles

Air is pulled down into the lungs by the action of two muscles. The **diaphragm** is a huge muscle, like a tent, which lies above the stomach and below the lungs. When it contracts it pulls itself downwards, making the chest cavity bigger. At the same time **muscles between the ribs** all shorten, and this widens the chest cavity. The result is a much larger space, with lower air pressure which pulls fresh air in, rather like British weather!

Being overweight, pregnant or having a large meal can restrict the movement of the diaphragm. When we have difficulty breathing we use accessory muscles such as those in the neck and shoulders to help us.

The amount of air we breathe

The average adult takes in about half a litre (1 pint) of air at each breath and takes twelve breaths per minute. Many people with respiratory disease have a device called a **peak flow spirometer**, which measures the maximum they can breathe out, and herbalists use these to monitor their patient's progress. Breathing in is an active process – muscles contract to enlarge the chest cavity. Breathing out is passive – muscles are not stimulated but relaxed. It is more difficult to breathe out if the airways are obstructed as there is no muscular force behind the movement.

The lungs

The lungs consist of millions of tiny sacs called **alveoli**, where oxygen diffuses into the blood and carbon dioxide is released from it via contact with minute, thin-walled blood vessels called **capillaries** which culminate in larger, very elastic blood vessels – the **pulmonary arteries** and **veins**. When oxygen diffuses into the blood stream, it is picked up by red blood cells, which contain **haemoglobin**. Carbon dioxide is largely dissolved in the blood directly as bicarbonate.

Insufficient oxygen or haemoglobin may cause breathlessness, as the lungs work harder to respond to the body's oxygen shortage. Each lung is encased in a fluid-lined sac called a **pleura**. Inflammation of this sac gives rise to the painful infective condition known as **pleurisy**.

Lymph drainage

Surrounding the respiratory organs are chains of **lymph nodes** and **ducts** which provide immune cells and drain infections from the area. You will often notice painful nodes in your neck, armpits and along the collarbone when you have a chest infection.

Nervous control of breathing

Breathing is largely controlled by a special group of nerve cells in the lower part of the brain which is sensitive to changes in oxygen and carbon dioxide levels. They relay messages to spinal nerves which control muscle movement in this area. This is what is called an **autonomic activity** – it happens without our being conscious of it. Nevertheless we can control breathing for a little while by holding our breath, breathing deeply and slowly as part of an exercise or examination. This control is exerted via the **vagus nerve**, which connects the lungs with our conscious centres in the brain cortex.

The effect of anxiety on breathing

Interconnections between the vagus nerve and other nerves can allow emotions to influence breathing, for example fear or anxiety can cause us to breathe faster. Prolonged anxiety can raise tension in muscles including those which are involved in breathing. This may limit movement of the diaphragm and rib muscles and worsen the bronchial spasm involved in asthma. These effects are caused by interactions of two groups of nervous messenger chemicals – **parasympathetic** in the vagus nerve and **sympathetic** in the spinal nerves.

Nervous messengers

When you are under emotional stress, or you are exercising strenuously, the body mobilises sympathetic nervous chemical messengers which cause:

- faster breathing rate
- dilation of bronchi

- extra blood flow to arm and leg muscles
- faster heart rate
- and decrease of digestive functions.

This is called the **fight or flight syndrome**.
Parasympathetic nerve messengers cause:

- greater digestive secretion and movement
- slower heart and breathing rate
- and constriction of bronchial tubes.

Chronic tension

Chronic tension and anxiety can lead to prolonged
excessive sympathetic stimulation of nerve endings in the
respiratory system, although the constricting effect of
irritants seems to prevent broncho-dilation which you
might expect from sympathetic nervous action.

Breathing habits

Patterns of breathing are to some extent learnt and
become a habit, for example shallow breathing or stooped
posture which inhibits muscular movement. Many
therapeutic exercise programmes for asthma and
bronchitis, such as yoga and the Buteyko method, try to
create new patterns of breathing.

Links with the circulatory system

The respiratory system is closely linked to the circulatory

system, especially the heart, as blood passes directly from the heart to the lungs before it is circulated around the body. Extra effort in breathing, and changes in pressure due to obstructions, place a strain on the heart. Reduced air-intake leads to oxygen deprivation in body tissues including the heart as blood fails to deliver its most vital supply. Heart problems can also affect breathing, for example cardiac asthma where fluid congests the lungs and causes coughing, especially at night.

Links with the digestive system

The vagus nerve also provides connections between the digestive organs and the respiratory system. Herbalists use these to apply herbal actions indirectly to the airways. You will read about these in Chapter 3.

Herbal help for other respiratory diseases

There are a number of respiratory conditions such as cystic fibrosis, emphysema and occupational lung diseases (farmer's lung, miner's lung, pigeon fancier's lung!) which benefit from using herbs, but they are outside the scope of this book. Use the Sources and Resources to find a local herbalist who can advise you.

Asthma explained

Asthma is an ancient Greek word which means panting. This respiratory disease has a number of features:

- Rapid, shallow, gasping breathing occurs because the bronchioles (small airways in the lungs) are constricted or become swollen, preventing air from reaching the alveoli.

- Breathing rate increases – panting – in response to oxygen deficiency and a sense of suffocation occurs because expiration (breathing out) is also impeded.

- Swelling of the mucous membrane occurs with secretion of thick, sticky mucus, in response to irritation by allergens or chemical irritants. Muscles in the bronchial walls contract, causing constriction as a defence mechanism to prevent further invasion.

- Cough reflexes are stimulated by mucus and irritants, especially when demand for oxygen is higher, and bronchi dilate, for example on exercise.

- Wheezing is heard as air is expired through narrowed airways, like blowing through a whistle.

- Obstruction by plugs of sticky mucus, which is so thick it cannot be passed by the ciliary hairs, may prevent normal breathing, resulting in severe breathlessness.

Causes of asthma

It appears that the potential to suffer from asthma is inherited. People who have **allergic** asthma, also called **atopic asthma** react to a number of allergens – rarely just one. Atopic asthma is usually worse in the summer, when pollen is circulating in the air. Atopic individuals often have other allergic conditions such as eczema.

Those who show no allergic tendency, sometimes called **bronchitic asthmatics**, are worse off in the winter, when infections are more common and cold air stimulates bronchospasm.

Both groups find that respiratory infections lead to increased swelling, mucus secretion and spasmodic coughing, which make their asthma worse.

Although the tendency to asthma and atopy is thought to be hereditary, environmental factors trigger the response. These include:

- tobacco and bonfire smoke
- animal dander, including wool
- pollen and fungal spores
- toiletries – hairspray, perfume etc
- industrial chemicals, including plastics
- petrol fumes
- drugs, including aspirin
- foods.

It is also known that anger and shock can trigger asthma attacks, as the breathing rate is increased and bronchial dilation allows irritants into the bronchial tree.

Increased incidence of asthma

It appears that asthma is increasing. One recent survey

showed that one in five schoolchildren at secondary schools has an inhaler. There are a number of possible explanations for this phenomenon.

Car fumes

It is possible that the different type of air pollution we experience in cities (car fumes rather than coal fire fumes) has caused a shift from bronchitis to asthma in common respiratory diseases. Some researchers have found that car petrol contains nitrogen compounds which paralyse the ciliary hairs in mucous membranes. This may allow irritants and allergens to penetrate the deeper airways, producing an asthmatic response in susceptible individuals. This is thought to happen inside the car as well as outside and is not affected by currently available filters and converters.

Carpeting

Another possible explanation for the increase in reported atopy is the rise in wall-to wall carpeting over the last 30 years. Once a futuristic luxury, this is now a normal purchase for the house. This type of flooring is thought to raise the amount of dust mites, animal and human dander we are exposed to at home, as it is trapped even in well vacuumed carpet. This belief has led to a growth in wood and laminate flooring as a 'hypo-allergenic alternative'.

On the other hand most people nowadays vacuum regularly, so it might be argued that there is less dust in modern houses than in the days when the carpet sweeper reigned supreme or when carpets were beaten once a year.

Central heating

Some people blame central heating for contributing to the rise in asthma, as the constant dry warmth prevents humidification of air and dries the mucous membrane, which prevents cilia from moving freely. It is, however, also thought that cold, damp houses too trigger asthma and bronchitis in children.

Synthetic compounds

Some researchers think that the amount of plastic and synthetic chemicals in our households are partly responsible for the rise in asthma, from nylon carpets to cleaning fluids and washing powders. They argue that our sensitive airways respond to these unnatural compounds with as much irritation as to natural allergens.

Bottle feeding

Research has shown that babies who are not breast-fed develop more of the sort of immunoglobulins which are involved in allergic reactions. An increase in bottle-fed babies could account for the increase in atopy. Further research is needed to confirm this, as many breast-fed babies also develop asthma, so additional factors may be involved.

Dietary causes

Many alternative practitioners suggest that some foods, such as cows' milk, are responsible for asthma and eczema. Direct food allergy causes have not been proved by current research although it is possible for food allergens to reach the bronchi via the blood stream, especially in those with damaged digestive linings (leaky gut syndrome). It is more likely that an imbalance of nutrients, such as plant oils and animal fats, may affect the outcome of an allergic asthmatic tendency. Guidelines on foods to increase and foods to use with caution for asthma and bronchitis are given in Chapter 6.

One last explanation for the rise in asthma may be that, as we see in crime statistics, more cases are reported than before, as more people visit their doctor for minor complaints such as a persistent cough and expect a prescription for treatment. To prescribe means to diagnose.

Bronchitis explained

Bronchitis is inflammation of the bronchial tubes. It involves:

- Swelling of the mucous membrane. This narrows the

airway, reducing the amount of air which can reach the alveoli.

- Over-secretion of mucous often thick and infected, which further obstructs the airways and prevents expiration.

- Air entrapment in the alveoli, causing disruption and destruction of their walls. This is known as emphysema, it sometimes occurs without preceding bronchitis. Together bronchitis and emphysema are known as **chronic obstructive airways disease**, **COAD** for short.

- Coughing – the cough reflex is triggered by the irritability of the mucous membrane and excess mucus.

- Breathlessness, even on mild exertion such as going upstairs. Insufficient oxygen reaches the alveoli and the sufferer often has to stop to get their breath.

Causes of bronchitis
- tobacco smoking
- industrial chemicals
- urban smog
- infections.

Apart from infections, which may cause an isolated episode of bronchitis, these factors cause damage on repeated exposure, rather than triggering attacks, as in asthma.

Incidence of bronchitis

Chronic bronchitis may not be as common nowadays for a number of reasons:

- more stringent health and safety regulations at work, which control exposure to pollutants
- effective antibiotic treatment for chest infections
- better – warmer, drier, more spacious – housing
- clean air laws controlling coal fire emissions (until 1963, when smokeless fuel was introduced, intense smogs and fogs were a regular feature of British winters).

∞ 2 ∞

What conventional
medicine can offer

Conventional treatment is aimed at keeping the airways
open, by:

- increasing bronchial dilation
- reducing inflammation
- and defeating bacterial infections.

In severe cases oxygen is provided to maintain adequate
blood concentration during a crisis. Pharmaceutical
preparations are provided for use at home in inhalation
devices which spread finely powdered dry material, or
dissolved in liquid (aerosols) into the throat. This method
of application concentrates most of the drug in the
airways, but some is absorbed into the blood, especially
with higher doses. It is possible that over-frequent use
might increase systemic absorption. The inhalant drugs
are also available in tablet form, but this allows them to
be absorbed systemically – reaching all other body tissues
via the bloodstream. Hospital and emergency treatment
may involve a nebuliser. This is a powered device which
reduces the drug to an even finer spray and pumps it into
the airways.

You may be prescribed the following:

- Bronchodilators:
  - B$_2$ adrenoceptor stimulants
  - anti-muscarinic bronchodialators.
- Methylxanthines.
- Combination bronchodilators.
- Adrenoceptor stimulants.
- Corticosteriods.
- Sodium cromoglycate.
- Antibiotics.
- Expectorants.

Bronchodilators

Bronchodilators work on the muscles of the bronchial tubes, keeping them maximally open.
There are different types, classified according to their length of action.

B$_2$ adrenoceptor stimulants

Those which produce short-term effects – 3-5 hours:

- salbutamol (brand names Ventolin, Volmax, Avomir)
- terbutaline (brand name Bricanyl)
- fenoterol (brand name Berotec).

Those which produce long-term effects – up to 12 hours:

- salmeterol (brand name Serevent)

- eformoterol (brand names Foradil, Oxis).

How they work

B_2 adrenoceptors are nerve cells found in the muscles of the bronchioles and bronchi. They receive messages from the sympathetic nervous system to allow muscles to relax, thus widening the bronchial tubes. Salbutamol mimics the nerve transmission which normally stimulates these receptors. In most people the bronchial tubes are almost maximally dilated all the time. The parasympathetic nervous system sends messages to constrict bronchial muscle and secrete mucus when irritated, to prevent further penetration of irritants and remove them. Asthma sufferers have chronically constricted airways due to this mechanism and immune responses. Extra stimulation of B_2 receptors is thought to override these parasympathetic messages and relax muscle, resulting in dilation.

Disadvantages

Salbutamol also stimulates nerve receptors in heart muscle, making it beat faster. It increases the urinary excretion of potassium, so can lead to muscle cramps. It is noted for causing a fine tremor, and a sense of emotional tension and headache, due to stimulating receptors in muscles and blood vessels. These effects are more associated with tablet use than inhalation, as little diffuses into the bloodstream with normal use of inhalers.

Concern has been expressed that bronchodilators could

make asthma worse and increase chest infections by allowing irritants to penetrate deeper into the bronchial tree. There is no research evidence for this but it is possible that the course of asthma may be prolonged by use of inhalers.

Anti-muscarinic bronchodilators

These are mainly used in bronchitis but are often prescribed with salbutamol. They are mainly inhaled.

- ipratropium (brand name Atrovent)
- oxytropium (brand name Oxivent).

How they work

These bronchodilating drugs act on parasympathetic nerve receptors in bronchial muscle, preventing their constricting action and reducing the secretion of mucus.

Disadvantages

The main side-effect is an increase in glaucoma a serious eye condition, especially where these drugs are used with B_2 stimulants such as salbutamol. Anyone with a family history of glaucoma who is taking these drugs should be monitored regularly by an optician.

Methylxanthines

This is a family of chemicals including caffeine and

theophylline which are found in tea, coffee and cocoa. They are given in tablet form for severe asthma, sometimes injected into a vein in acute cases.

How they work

Methylxanthines act on nerve receptors in bronchial muscle, causing it to relax and dilate. In the right dose they are supposed to cause this effect without affecting other organs such as the heart, brain, blood vessels and kidneys, which all have receptors for these chemicals.

Theophylline also inhibits the release of mast cells which are responsible for tissue swelling in allergy.

Disadvantages

This medicine causes increase in heart rate (tachycardia) and disturbance in regularity (arythmia) as well as high blood pressure, liver problems and potassium deficiency. You may notice symptoms such as headache, palpitations, nausea, insomnia and irritability if your dose exceeds the therapeutic level. Much the same happens with excessive use of tea, which has one saving grace – it contains potassium!

Regular tea drinking would add to the effect of theophylline. When one medicine or herb does this to another, it is known as **potentiation**. Many British people drink a litre of tea a day and wouldn't think of reporting this to their doctor as a medicine.

Combination bronchodilators

Anti-muscarinics and B_2 adrenoceptor stimulants are often combined. For example:

- fenoterol
- ipratropium (brand names Duovent, Combivent).

Adrenoceptor stimulants

Some of these chemicals are derived from the plant kingdom, and some are based on human neuro-chemicals. For example:

- ephedrine
- adrenaline
- orciprenaline (brand name Alupent).

How they work

Adrenoceptor stimulants stimulate nerve receptors in bronchial muscle walls and mucosal linings, causing sympathetic nervous actions. This helps to reduce mucosal swelling as well as secretion and dilates the bronchi. Ephedrine is available over the counter as Sudafed. Adrenaline is used in acute allergic reactions (anaphylaxis).

Disadvantages

Because of sympathetic effects on receptors in the brain,

digestive and circulatory systems, these drugs cause rapid heart beat, dry mouth, high blood pressure, cold hands and feet, anxiety, insomnia and restlessness. If you have used Sudafed you may have noticed some of these stimulant effects which stop when you cease taking it.

Corticosteroids

These are prescribed for asthma to reduce inflammation. They can be inhaled and are frequently given in pill form. For example:

- beclometasone dipropionate (brand names Aerobec, Becotide, Qvar, Becloforte, Ventride)
- budenoside (brand name Pulmicort)
- fluticasone propionate (brand names Seretide, Flixotide).

How they work

Corticosteroids prevent immune cells from making interleukins – chemicals which connect parts of the immune system in the process of inflammation. They inhibit the production of prostaglandins and leukotrienes – inflammatory chemicals especially involved in swelling and vasodilation. Corticosteroids also reduce the number of immune cells.

Disadvantages

This group of drugs has a number of ill effects which happen because they alter protein synthesis in body cells. Structures such as muscle, skin and bone become thin and growth is affected in children. Immunity is less effective because of the reduction in immune cell synthesis. These side-effects are not entirely eliminated by only using inhalers, although greatly diminished if small doses for short periods are used.

Sodium cromoglycate

This is prescribed for allergic asthmas as an inhalant aerosol and is also available in combination with salbutamol. For example:

- sodium cromoglycate (brand name Intal)
- salbutamol and sodium cromoglycate (brand name Aerocrom).

How it works

Sodium cromoglycate suppresses chemicals released when allergens meet anti-bodies including histamine and leukotrienes. This action reduces swelling in allergic asthma, but it has to be applied directly as the allergen is present; it has no effect later.

Disadvantages

It has practically no side effects, its disadvantage is that it has such a limited application, having no effect in non-allergic asthma.

Antibiotics

These may be prescribed for asthmatics who suffer chest infections but are more commonly prescribed for bronchitis sufferers. There is a large number of different products, only those most commonly prescribed for respiratory problems are mentioned here.

Penicillins:
- ampicillin (brand name Penbritin)
- amoxycillin (brand name Amoxil).

Broad spectrum anti-biotics:
- tetracycline (brand name Achromycin)
- erythromycin (brand name Erymax).

How they work

Antibiotics interfere with the cell walls of a number of bacteria, which causes their destruction. The broad spectrum antibiotics are so-called because they affect a wider range of bacteria than other antibiotics.

Disadvantages

These disadvantages apply to all antibiotics. They reduce the number of enzymes and the whole bacterial population of the human gut, which are known as 'friendly bacteria' because they live in balance with each other and may perform useful functions. This can result in thrush and diarrhoea which may linger after stopping treatment.

Penicillin is noted for causing hyper-sensitivity reactions such as swelling, sickness, joint pain and high temperatures. Being water-soluble it can irritate the kidneys.

A wider concern is over-use and increasing resistance to these antibiotics, which results in less effective drugs and fewer choices for patients.

Expectorants

There is only one expectorant prescribed, ammonia and ipecacuanha mixture. Its entry in the British National Formulary is accompanied by comment that facilitated expectoration is a myth and that expectorants work by placebo effect (where the patient experiences improvement due to his belief that the medicine will work). A full page of over-the counter expectorant preparations follows, which is presumably offered as proof of public fallibility. Herbalists take a different view of expectorants so these will be covered thoroughly in the next chapter.

∼ 3 ∼

Using herbs to treat asthma and bronchitis

Herbal approaches will include taking herbal medicine as well as using inhalants regularly. Methods for preparing these are given in Chapter 5. Herbal medicine is the leading alternative to conventional pharmaceutical treatment. When herbalists make up a prescription for patients with asthma and bronchitis problems, they take into account all the factors which contribute to their health and try to improve all the systems which are affected by respiratory difficulties. This is called a wholistic approach. It is the main difference between conventional and herbal treatment. In addition to prescribing herbal medicine, herbalists would want a patient to start exercises and dietary changes in a strategy to maintain general well-being.

Aims of herbal treatment

- Relieve infections and strengthen immunity using immuno-stimulants and anti-infectives.
- Reduce swelling and obstruction – using anti-inflammatories.

- Relax respiratory muscles – using muscle relaxants.
- Increase elimination of mucus – using expectorants.
- Improve circulation – using circulatory tonics.
- Improve digestion and nutrition – using digestive tonics and plant foods.
- Reduce allergic response – using anti - allergenics.
- Relieve emotional tension – using nervine relaxants.

How herbs work

Balanced constituents

Herbs contain small quantities of chemicals compared to modern pharmaceutical products which extract or synthesise one chemical in much larger amounts to obtain an effect. This means there is no danger of sudden physiological changes which cause side-effects. Most herbs contain a large number of active constituents which work together to create one or more effects. The more we find out about herbs, the more we realise that each constituent is a valued part of the whole. Negative effects are balanced by positive ones.

A good example of the balance within many herbs is found in St John's wort. Recently much has been made of a research trial which showed that a St John's wort preparation made liver enzymes more active, which reduced the effect of other drugs taken at the time. Although this trial didn't examine women taking the pill, it was assumed that this effect would extend to the oral contraceptive pill. The St John's wort preparation used in this trial was standardised to contain a larger amount of one constituent, hypericin, than all the others. Not only has hypericin failed to show anti-depressant activity on its own, in repeated trials, but another constituent, hyperforin, has been shown to counterbalance hypericin in its effect on liver enzymes. Many other research trials on St John's wort have shown no adverse effect on drugs taken simultaneously and doctors in Germany continue to prescribe it as a relaxing anti-depressant.

In Britain doctors are advised to warn their patients that their oral contraception may not be safe if they take St John's wort and herbalists caution patients to use non-standardised forms of this herb in moderate quantities if they are taking medication with a 'narrow therapeutic range' (where small alterations in dose make big differences in effect). There is no direct evidence that St John's wort affects the contraceptive pill and no reported cases of pregnancy while combining them, but NIMH members would advise patients who are worried about this to use extra contraceptive methods or change to another herbal remedy.

Synergy

Similar bad publicity surrounds liquorice, where a constituent called glycyrrhizin is thought to raise blood pressure, but in fact dozens of other constituents act to lower it, in particular by diuresis (elimination of water).

Where two or more constituents act together to create the same effect, this is known as synergy.

Some herbs, like garlic, contain several ingredients which provide help for our circulation on multiple levels. Its antibiotics protect against infection and repair the damage caused by wear and tear on the insides of our blood vessels. Digestive stimulants help the absorption of sugars and fats from the bloodstream. As a circulatory tonic it reduces the stickiness of platelets, dilates the capillaries, causes mild sweating and increases kidney activity, so helps to protect against strokes, lowers blood pressure and helps to protect the heart from strain in exercise. This type of multiple activity is a feature of many herbs which enable them to support the wholistic approach very well.

Slow, cumulative action

Although some herbs act swiftly, like the sleep-inducer, valerian, herbal remedies generally act slowly and their effects are cumulative. They gently rebalance physiological processes, as though switch after switch is thrown until the full effect is achieved. This can take weeks, sometimes months, but it is worth waiting for, as the risk of side effects is very low, due to the tiny amounts of chemicals involved. Valerian appears to improve the quality of your sleep as well as helping you to doze off and doesn't cause a sluggish feeling in the morning, because the chemicals it contains are in small amounts and are cleared from the body fairly quickly. This lower level of activity may be disappointing if you want to be 'knocked out', but using herbs like valerian as part of a plan to restore sleep patterns can be effective.

How do herbal remedies get to their target?

Herbal compounds need to be absorbed across the wall of the digestive tract, so they have to be released from their structures (stem, root, leaf, flower or berry etc.) first of all. Hot water and alcohol do some of this job for us, so that teas and tinctures are more easily absorbed than tablets and capsules, which need to be broken down physically before the active chemicals are separated from the inert matter to which they are attached. All food and medicine passes through the liver (in the blood circulation) before it finally enters the body tissues, where it is used.

Sometimes chemical compounds need help in crossing through the wall of the digestive tract into the blood stream. Carrier chemicals can be attached to compounds and ferry them through channels in the gut lining. Hydrochloride is frequently found to be part of conventional drug names as it has this function.

Do herbs have any advantages over modern drugs?

Herbal compounds often have an advantage over synthesised chemicals in some respects. They have naturally occurring carrier chemicals already attached to them. These are often in the sugar family. Some are known as glycosides and these and their relatives, monosaccharides, are attracting a lot of interest in the modern research world. These carrier chemicals enable herbal compounds to enter target cells more easily, and may explain how herbs can have an effect, even at quite low doses. This is what is meant by affinity. Herbs are said to have a greater affinity for the human body, like spare parts dedicated to a particular engine made by the same manufacturer. Herbs contain many different chemicals in small quantities, so the risk of side-effects is low compared with the very strong effects of single chemicals in orthodox medicine.

Are herbs safe?

All the herbs which British Herbalists use are safe when used in the correct dose for the right ailment. The herbs mentioned in this book have been selected for their safety in untrained hands, although you may need professional help with your diagnosis. The National Institute of Medical Herbalists (NIMH) – see page 140 maintains an extensive data bank and works with government watchbodies to ensure safety of its herbs. Recently some attention was given to the group of compounds called pyrrolizidine alkaloids, present in several plants including comfrey, because they can cause (reversible) damage to the liver if ingested in large quantities. The evidence on comfrey is not based on human case studies and the research involved feeding rats exclusively on large amounts of comfrey. There is only one reported case of human toxicity world-wide, which concerned a woman who took comfrey tea many times a day concurrently with illegal drugs in high doses over a long period. Several governments, including that of Britain, made moves to ban its use. After extensive discussions with the NIMH, it was agreed to limit use to the guidelines given above, and restrict the root (which contains more PAs) to external use only. In this way herbalists acknowledge the potential risk and demonstrate the history of safe use.

The constituents of herbs

Another advantage of herbal medicine is that there are so many different plants with similar actions, but different combinations or constituents. You can change from one to another to avoid becoming tolerant or developing sensitivities. For example, there are many anti-inflammatory herbs, each with their own supplementary actions including hormonal, diuretic, anti-spasmodic and relaxing effects. Herbs may act on several different aspects of a condition at the same time, like garlic which provides help for our circulation on several levels. As an antibiotic, it repairs the damage caused by wear and tear on the insides of our blood vessels. As a digestive stimulant it helps the absorption of sugars and fats from the bloodstream. As a circulatory tonic it reduces the stickiness of platelets, dilates the capillaries, causes mild sweating and increases kidney activity, so it helps to protect against strokes and lowers blood pressure slightly.

Combining herbs with orthodox medication

Some drugs are altered by liver enzymes, so that they enter the main blood circulation in a different form. Some herbs (especially **bitters**) stimulate the liver cells to work harder, or cause more liver cells to be active and this can affect other drugs because the liver removes them from circulation before they have had a chance to do their work. Digoxin is one of these and is also a drug with a 'narrow therapeutic window'. This means that the difference between an insufficient, a beneficial and a harmful dose is very small, so that small changes in the amount getting through to the bloodstream may result in the drug not working as it should. Two other drugs like this are Cyclosporin, used to prevent transplant rejection, and Phenytoin, an anti-epileptic. It is very important to check with a qualified herbalist and let your doctor know if you are adding herbal medicine to medication you are currently using.

There are many herbs which can be taken safely with other medicines, so don't feel deterred from trying, but do seek professional advice. Herbs can be used to offset the side effects of necessary medication, like indigestion or nausea. They may enable you to take less of a remedy which you need, but which has troublesome side-effects.

The important thing is how you feel, and that you don't endanger your health. It may be simple to ask your doctor to monitor blood levels of drugs and adjust the dose if necessary.

It would not be wise to embark on herbal medicine without medical supervision if you are on anti-psychotic medication, as you may not be aware that your mental condition has deteriorated when your current medication ceases to work. You may have strong feelings about the disadvantages of your drugs, but may not realise how your behaviour is changing and affecting others badly. It is possible to have herbal medicine for other complaints while on medication for psychosis, but you must consult your doctor first and allow yourself to be monitored.

If you are on chemotherapy for cancer, it would be better to wait until your treatment has finished before taking herbal medicine, unless you are looking for help with troublesome side effects such as nausea or diarrhoea. Several herbs can help here without reducing the effectiveness of your anti-cancer drugs.

Drugs to be careful with	*Conditions to be careful with*
Anti-arhythmics	Pregnancy
Anti-epileptics	Epilepsy
Anti-psychotics	Schizophrenia, psychosis
Immune suppressants	Organ transplant
Anti-cancer drugs	Allergies

Sometimes over the counter herbal medicines are labelled with contraindications. This is required by law in Germany. It means for example that you will be told if you shouldn't take the medicine if you are pregnant, taking another specific medication, have an allergy or a certain medical condition. This will become more common in Europe in the future.

The advantages of using whole plant preparations

Although there are variations between plants around the world, herbalists believe that plants would only have gained a historical reputation for certain effects if their constituents were robust enough to maintain the same effect wherever they were grown or whatever minor differences there might be between local plant populations. Rosemary is distinctively rosemary whether it's grown on a London balcony or in a Caribbean back yard. If only one variety in one particular year made someone feel better, its reputation would not have stood the test of time.

The current trend, based on scientific research, is to standardise the process of growing, harvesting and storing herbs, so that their use is sustainable and patients get the best value from them. Medical herbalists also recommend using whole, unaltered preparations, as nature presented them, so that each constituent is represented in natural amounts. This is the type of preparation on which traditional knowledge is based and which you will be able to make at home. Don't forget that smell and taste are still very reliable indicators of the effectiveness of herbal medicine. It is also useful to remember that people vary much more than plants do!

Herbal applications

Herbal applications include a number of approaches, both conventional and unconventional, such as:

- expectorants
- anti-inflammatories
- antibacterials
- anti-spasmodics or anti-tussives
- bronchodilators and decongestants
- immuno-stimulants
- emollients
- anti-allergenics
- circulatory tonics
- bitter digestive tonics.

Expectorants

This group contains a large number of herbs with slightly different actions. Expectorants are meant to increase the clearance of thick mucus from the lungs and bronchial tree. Their name derives from Latin, *ex* = out of, *pectoris* =

chest. There have been several articles in the popular press and medical journals stating that expectorants don't work. There is little clinical evidence to back this claim up but a fair amount of acceptable theory and plenty of traditional evidence that they do work. It is likely that anti-inflammatory, antibacterial and emollient herbs are also called expectorants by older herbalists, as we find these actions under this general term which appears to include all herbs which 'clear' the chest.

There are two main sorts of expectorant – stimulating and relaxing.

Stimulating expectorants

These are thought to increase the cough reflex and ciliary beating by acting on the stomach wall, although there is some discussion as to whether this reflex stimulation really occurs. They are usually able to cause vomiting in larger doses. Ipecacuanha, still available on prescription, belongs to this group and some, like squills, are found in commercially available cough remedies. They are not popular with herbalists now, but may repay some more clinical and theoretical research. They are not discussed in this book as they are not suitable for home prescribing.

Relaxing expectorants

This group includes all those herbs which don't stimulate the stomach lining, but includes those which stimulate the secretion of thin mucus. Many herbs which contain saponins appear to do this, possibly by changing the walls and activity of mucus-producing cells. Some aromatic herbs do this by directly irritating the linings of the airways when inhaled.

Anti-inflammatories

Inflammation in the airways involves swelling and over-secretion of thickened mucus.

Herbal anti-inflammatories for the respiratory system reduce swelling, irritability and secretion of sticky mucus. They may achieve this by interfering in the process of immune defence, preventing antigen-antibody complexes from summoning chemicals such as histamine, which allow liquid to leak from cells into spaces between tissues. This relieves swelling quickly. Some anti-inflammatories prevent the production of inflammatory chemicals such as prostaglandins.

Antibacterials

Antibacterials destroy small invading organisms such as bacteria but they generally don't work on small viruses. Each antibacterial reacts with a specific range of bacteria, some affect a larger range than others. These are like broad spectrum antibiotics, but herbs do not destroy as many bacteria as pharmaceutical preparations. This can be an advantage in mild infections if the dose is repeated regularly as herbal antibacterials are thought to allow natural defence cells (normally also destroyed by antibiotics) to survive and build up a response. This slow, gentle approach may be very suitable for repeated infections and it has the added benefit of sparing digestive enzymes, which are also destroyed by conventional antibiotics. Sometimes they are referred to as anti-infectives because of this 'background level' of anti-bacterial activity.

Anti-spasmodic or anti-tussives

Anti-spasmodics relieve excess muscular tension and activity by reducing the number of messages which are received in bronchial muscles from the brain or by reducing further transmission of messages directly in the muscle. They are also known as peripheral relaxants.

Anti-tussives means cough relieving. Anti-tussives may be anti-spasmodics or emollients (see below).

Bronchodilatora and decongestants

These are explained in the conventional medicines section. Herbal bronchodilators such as datura are not available over the counter, as they are classified as Schedule 3 herbs. This is list of herbs, agreed by the National Institute of Medical Herbalists and the government during the drafting of the British Medicines Act of 1968, which have some dangerous properties and may only be dispensed as part of a consultation.

Immuno-stimulants

These are also referred to as anti-infectives, as they increase resistance to infections. Some, like echinacea, are very well researched. It has been shown that they act by increasing the number of immune cells, and by facilitating their action, making bacteria more 'sticky' or more recognisable to our immune defences. They can make immune cells such as macrophages and interleukins more effective. There is no evidence of these herbs increasing auto-immunity or allergic tendency. More research is needed to establish just how many herbs have this important action as herbalists suspect that there may be many more which have not been researched yet.

Aromatic herbs

It is possible that aromatic compounds in herbs such as thyme, pine, rosemary etc remain in the body tissues to aid defence against infection. This theory is popular in France, where they talk about the *terrain* which aromatics defend.

Anti-virals

Many herbalists also think that plants such as vervein, lemon balm and St John's wort have some type of anti-viral effect, although it is not confirmed by research yet. It is possible that their anti-depressant effect confers strength on the immune system. There is evidence to show that depressed individuals have lowered immunity – fewer

white blood cells etc. This is a very exciting area for
further research.

Emollients

These are also called demulcents in many herbals. They
may assist expectoration by reducing muscular spasm.
This is achieved by action on the stomach and
oesophagus. Nervous stimulation is inhibited by reflex in
the respiratory airways as messages travel in the nerve arcs.
Most emollients contain soothing mucilage, a starchy
substance which reduces inflammatory irritation on
contact. Some emollients also contain saponins, so may
be working to free the airways in two different ways at
once. Where a herb also has antibacterial properties it may
be classified as a pectoral (chest) tonic. Some emollients
such as Benzoin, contain resins which act on exposed
surfaces directly when they are inhaled.

Anti-allergenics

Anti-allergenic herbs work by reducing some of the effects
of the antigen-antibody meeting. The effects are not well
defined but some herbs such as chamomile, and possibly
elderflower and nettle, are known to reduce the number of
mast cells and prevent them from secreting substances
which are involved in swelling and allergic reactions.
These actions are rarely recorded in traditional herbals,
although a better understanding of mucous membrane
tonics might reveal more anti-allergenic action.

Circulatory tonics

These herbs increase blood flow by dilating blood vessels and this helps to create general health as well as improving the function of specific organs. Traditionally plasters made with pungent herbs were applied to the chest to increase blood flow in cases of infection, and vapour rubs are still sold with this type of ingredient. Many cough remedies based on traditional remedies contain pungent herbs such as chilli, for a similar effect. There is no modern research to show if this approach is helpful in chronic chest conditions.

Bitter digestive tonics

These work by stimulating digestive secretions in the mouth, stomach, pancreas and liver. Bitters are noted for their action on the liver, increasing bile flow which emulsifies fats and transports excess from the bloodstream. Pungent herbs (hot spices) irritate linings which respond by increased secretion of digestive enzymes. These break down starch, fat and protein as well as transporting essential vitamins and minerals across the gut wall into the blood circulation. Aromatic herbs stimulate the digestive tract in a similar way, though more gently, and they reduce bacterial fermentation which causes wind and colic.

Digestive tonics usually also contain bitters. The aromatic bitters are well known as part of the British cookery tradition, especially in association with meat dishes. They were the mainstay of herbal manufacturers years ago. 'Tonic bitters' were sold in every pharmacy, and 'tonic stout ' was prescribed on the NHS for elderly patients as well as breastfeeding mums by doctors until the early 1970s. Many of the famous herbal tonics are still based on bitters and nearly every country has a national favourite. The French drink Gentian wine, Swedes export their bitters, the British put theirs in stouts and beers, Italians prefer vermouth, Mexicans use angostura which gave us pink gin.

Bitter taste buds are located at the back of your tongue. They are designed to detect poisons and trigger a gag reflex, so you spit out food which is bad for you. Humans can overcome the bitter revulsion reflex by three methods: telling ourselves it's good for us, adding nice flavours or adding alcohol! The body however still working to the primeval instruction handbook, initiates a process to rid the body of unwanted chemicals. The liver produces more enzymes and bile in response to messages sent to the brain from the taste-buds. Saliva flows abundantly to cleanse the mouth, and activity in the stomach and pancreas increases, resulting in better absorption of nutrients and elimination of toxins. Pre-dinner drinks are good for you after all!

A recent hospital trial showed that patients who received nasty tasting medicine recovered more quickly than those whose medicine tasted bland. The effect was thought to be psychological, patients felt better because they thought their horrible medicine was more effective. Herbalists think that the bitter effect might have played a tonic role in this experiment.

Relaxants

Herbal relaxants relieve tension and restore nervous activity to a normal level, whereas sedatives reduce brain activity to below normal functioning level. This can improve concentration rather than impairing it, so it is a good example of a balancing action for which herbs are well known. These herbs work in two ways:

- Nervine relaxants act centrally, by reducing the brain's sensitivity to nerve messages from the periphery – skin, joints, muscles etc.
- Muscle relaxants act peripherally, on nerve centres in the spinal chord, or on nerve endings in the skin, reducing the number of messages sent from the periphery to the brain. They are also called anti-spasmodics.

Many herbs have both central and peripheral actions.

Wholistic therapies and breathing exercises

Herbs can help you to manage or overcome asthma and bronchitis, but you should also consider other therapies which improve breathing and increase relaxation. You could visit your local complementary medicine clinic's open day to find out more. Body and foot massage are noted for their relaxing effects and there is a type of therapy which involves drumming on the back, related to expectoration techniques in physiotherapy clinics in the 1950s and 60s in Britain.

Yoga

Yoga is a system of exercises developed over hundreds of years in India. Both meditational yoga and yoga for health- Hatha Yoga – include many exercises for breathing which help to regulate and deepen breathing as well as aiding expectoration. Some health professionals have noticed that children (and later adults) with asthma develop permanently shallow, open –mouthed, irregular breathing patterns which make their asthma worse. Yoga exercises can help these people overcome these breathing habits.

Buteyko

A Russian researcher called Buteyko has made lecture tours teaching his methods of 'retraining' breathing to severe asthma sufferers. He emphasises the importance of breathing through the nose and sometimes asks his subjects to apply sticking plaster to their mouths to prevent relapse into mouth- breathing. Yoga encourages this in a safer way by exercises in which one pinches first one nostril, then the other, alternately to draw air forcefully through each side of the nose. Establishing regular deep nasal breathing helps to discourage infections and reduce the constriction which causes asthmatic crises. Physiotherapists used to recommend swimming as a means of practising controlled breathing.

❧ 4 ❧

Directory of useful herbs

You will need to use a number of strategies to relieve asthma and bronchitis. Preventive approaches are covered in Chapter 6 on eating for a healthy respiratory system. You can use the information in this section to select the right herbs. The case histories in Chapter 7 guide you in building classic recipes or tailoring one to your own individual needs.

Herbs are usually categorised by their actions, and each herb will have some primary and some secondary actions. In some the actions are of equal importance. To treat asthma and bronchitis you may need expectorants, anti-inflammatories, antibacterials, anti-spasmodics, bronchodilators, immuno-stimulants, emollients, anti-allergenics, circulatory tonics, bitter digestive tonics and relaxants. When you read the case histories later, you will see how this directory can be used to pick herbs from the various categories.

EXPECTORANTS

Benzoin	Elecampane	Horehound
Cowslips	Hyssop	Thyme
Elderflower	Mullein	

Benzoin

Latin name	Styrax benzoin
Origin	Asia
Part used	Tree sap (gum)
Dose	1/2 teaspoon to 1/2 pint boiling water, inhaled 1-3 times daily, or essential oil heated as ambient vapour.
Constituents	Cinnamic, benzoic acid, benzaldehyde, vanillin
Primary actions	Expectorant Antibacterial
Secondary action	Anti-inflammatory
How it works	The sweet smelling acids are contained in a resin which melts in hot water, although the remains stick to the sides of the water vessel. They are antibacterial and soothing and penetrate deep into the airways as they are carried on steam.
Growing guide	Cannot be grown in Britain, requires tropical temperature.
Caution	Use an old cup or bowl as the resin sticks tenaciously to the sides. Surgical spirit will remove stubborn traces.

Cowslips

Latin name	Primula vera
Origin	Europe
Part used	Flowers
Dose	1/2 teaspoon per cup Tincture 2ml, 1-3 times daily

Constituents	Saponins, volatile oil, glycosides, flavonoids, phenols, tannins
Primary action	Expectorant
Secondary actions	Relaxant
	Anti-inflammatory
How it works	The saponins are thought to be responsible for the expectorant action, either by irritating the mucous membrane or by helping mucus cells release thin secretions by acting on their walls. Flavonoids are anti-inflammatory by stabilising the blood vessel walls so that leakiness and swelling are reduced. Flavonoids are also anti-spasmodic, which helps to relieve bronchial muscle tension. It isn't known which constituents have the sedative effect which is particularly noted in cowslip wine!
Growing guide	Cowslips can be easily grown from seed under glass and planted out in the spring. They like damp soil and will tolerate dappled shade.

Elderflower

Latin name	Sambucus niger
Origin	Europe
Part used	Flowers
Dose	1 teaspoon per cup
	Tincture 4ml, 1-3 times daily
Constituents	Volatile oil, ursolic acid, essential fatty acids, phenols, flavonoids, sterols

Primary actions	Anti-inflammatory
	Expectorant
Secondary action	Anti-spasmodic
How it works	Elderflower is the main ingredient in most herbal prescriptions for upper respiratory problems such as sinusitis, hayfever and colds. It is a useful addition to treatments for asthma and bronchitis. The ursolic acid is thought to provide the anti-inflammatory effects, possibly supported by the essential fatty acids which help to stabilise mucous cell walls, preventing leakage and inflammatory swelling. The phenols are mildly antibacterial and expectorant. Sterols may add to the expectorant effect.
Growing guide	Elderflower throws out suckers which have to be removed to achieve a single trunk. It can grow to about 15 feet over many years, and gives early white blossom for lemonade and glossy black berries for wine. The bark is corky and very attractive on an old tree. The common form is very underrated as a garden tree.

Elecampane

Latin name	Inula helenium
Origin	Europe
Part used	Root
Dose	1 teaspoon per cup
	Tincture 2ml, 1-3 times daily

Constituents	Inulin, helenin, volatile oil (including camphor), bitters, resins, saponins, mucilage, choline
Primary actions	Expectorant
	Anti-inflammatory
Secondary actions	Antibacterial
	Digestive tonic
How it works	The volatile oils and resins are strongly antibacterial and the saponins are thought to increase production of thin mucus which aids expectoration. The volatile oil contains camphor, which is decongestant by increasing the flow of mucus, and muscle relaxing. The mucilage, with helenin, provides a soothing, anti-inflammatory effect on the throat and by reflex from the digestive tract. It is possible that choline provides precursors for nerve transmittor chemicals which regulate heart and breathing rate as well as cell secretion, although the amount is tiny compared to that used in research trials.
Growing guide	A magnificent, 6-foot tall perennial with a huge yellow dandelion-like flower. Easily grown from seed under glass. The fresh root has a superb fragrance.

Horehound

Latin name	Marrubium vulgare
Origin	Europe
Part used	Leaf

Dose	1 teaspoon per cup
	Tincture 4ml, 1-3 times daily
Constituents	Bitters, volatile oil (including pinene, fenchene, camphor), mucilage, choline, alkaloids (including betonicine).
Primary actions	Expectorant
	Anti-inflammatory
Secondary actions	Anti-spasmodic
	Digestive tonic
How it works	Horehound contains bitter compounds which trigger secretion of digestive juices. This is responsible for its tonic effect. The volatile oil is antibacterial and anti-spasmodic. It is possible that choline provides precursors for neurotransmittors which regulate heart and breathing rate as well as cell secretion. Horehound has a traditional reputation for normalising arhythmic heart beat although the amount of choline is tiny compared with the amounts used to obtain effects in research trials. It may be a synergistic effect of the whole herb (see How Herbs Work page 38) The mucilage provides a soothing effect, acting on the throat and by reflex from the digestive tract.
Growing guide	An attractive, small, grey-leaved perennial plant which may be grown from seed under glass. Requires well-drained soil and sunny position.

Hyssop

Latin name	Hyssopus officinalis
Origin	Middle East
Part used	Leaf
Dose	1 teaspoon per cup
	Tincture 4ml, 1-3 times daily
Constituents	Volatile oil (including pinene, camphor), flavonoids
Primary actions	Expectorant
	Anti-spasmodic
Secondary actions	Anti-bacterial
	Anti-inflammatory
How it works	The volatile oil is both antibacterial and anti-spasmodic, helping to relieve muscular tension in asthma. Flavonoids are also anti-inflammatory by stabilising blood vessel walls, reducing leakage and swelling. Camphor is mildly decongestant by increasing the flow of thin mucus secretion. It also contributes an anti-spasmodic action and, by numbing surfaces to which it is applied directly, is mildly pain relieving. It has been used in rheumatic rubs and inhalant mixes for asthma and bronchitis.
Growing guide	A small perennial with intense blue flowers. Grow from seed under glass, plant in well-drained soil in a sunny spot.

Mullein

Latin name	Verbascum thapsus
Origin	Europe
Part used	Leaf
Dose	1 teaspoon per cup
	Tincture 4ml, 1-3 times daily
Constituents	Volatile oil, saponins, mucilage, flavonoids, glycosides (including aucubin)
Primary actions	Expectorant
	Anti-inflammatory
Secondary actions	Emollient
How it works	Saponins stimulate the mucous membranes, directly on inhaling and via the bloodstream, which increases the flow of thin mucus. This effect is apparently neutralised by our cholesterol after about a week, so mullein is best used in alternation with other remedies or for short courses. The flavonoids also stabilise blood vessel walls, which helps to reduce inflammatory swelling. Mucilage is emollient which reduces inflammation directly. The volatile oil is bactericidal but is present in very small amounts.
Growing guide	Grown from seed under glass. Plant out in a sunny spot with well drained soil. Mullein grows to a magnificent 8 feet, but doesn't spread, with beautiful, pale yellow spikes of flowers. Watch out for the equally beautiful mullein moth caterpillar! It has black and yellow stripes and can demolish leaves by the

	hour.
Caution	Strain the tea well as small hairs may remain from the leaves.

Thyme

Latin name	Thymus vulgaris
Origin	Europe
Part used	Leaf
Dose	1 teaspoon per cup
	Tincture 4ml, 1-3 times daily
Constituents	Volatile oil, phenols, flavonoids, saponins, bitters
Primary actions	Expectorant
	Antibacterial
Secondary actions	Anti-spasmodic
	Digestive tonic
How it works	Thyme's action is mainly due to its antibacterial volatile oil which is also anti-spasmodic. This helps to relax bronchial muscle. The flavonoids help to prevent small blood vessels from leaking, which reduces swelling. The volatile oil is also mildly irritant to mucous membranes, so increases flow of thin mucus. The bitters stimulate secretion of digestive juices, which provides the tonic effect. The saponins may also stimulate the free flow of mucus by acting on secretory cell walls.
Growing guide	Easy to grow from seed and small cuttings under glass. Needs a fairly sunny spot and

can be trimmed to make a small hedge, but needs replacing every three years as it becomes thin and woody.

ANTI-INFLAMMATORIES

Coltsfoot	Eyebright
Comfrey	Liquorice

Coltsfoot

Latin name	Tussilago farfara
Origin	Europe
Part used	Flowers
Dose	1 teaspoon per cup
	Tincture 4ml, 1-3 times daily (can also be smoked)
Constituents	Mucilage (polysaccharides), bitters, flavonoids, sterols, tannins, pyrrolizidine alkaloids.
Primary actions	Anti-inflammatory
	Expectorant
Secondary actions	Emollient
	Anti-spasmodic
	Immuno-stimulant
How it works	The mucilage is emollient and anti-inflammatory, both directly to the surface and by reflex from the digestive tract. Its polysaccharides are also thought to be responsible for the immuno-stimulant effect of the flowers (increasing phagocytic cell

action), which has been noted in clinical research. Flavonoids help to prevent inflammatory swelling by making blood vessels less leaky. It is not known exactly which constituents provide the sedative anti-spasmodic effect. The sterols may be responsible for its expectorant action. Pyrrolizidine alkaloids are noted for liver toxicity but there are very small amounts present in the flowers. Coltsfoot has been used for centuries in children's cough syrups with no reported ill-effects and recent research has confirmed that it is harmless in normal doses. There are no government concerns in Britain over its safety. Coltsfoot remains one of the most important herbs for respiratory illness.

Growing guide   Grown from seed directly sown in spring, or from rootlets pulled in autumn.

Comfrey

Latin name	Symphytum officinalis
Origin	Europe
Part used	Leaf
Dose	1 teaspoon per cup
	Tincture 4ml, 1-3 times daily
Constituents	Allantoin, mucilage, pyrrolizidine alkaloids, phenols, choline, tannins, bitters
Primary actions	Healing
	Anti-inflammatory

Secondary actions   Emollient
                      Astringent
How it works   Allantoin and mucilage are soothing and
                      healing, phenols are antibacterial. The whole
                      leaf tea stimulates production of anti-
                      inflammatory chemicals. The tannins are
                      astringent, toning tissues to which they are
                      directly applied, and antibacterial,
                      coagulating bacterial protein on direct
                      contact. Pyrrolizidine alkaloids are present in
                      small amounts in leaves and could cause
                      problems in long-term, high-dose use or in
                      cases of pre-existing liver disease.
Growing guide   Grow from root cuttings. Forms a large
                      clump 4ft high. Comfrey will tolerate heavy
                      soil and semi-shade.
Caution   Government guidelines in Britain, agreed
                      with the NIMH, recommend no more than 3
                      cups daily for no more than eight weeks.

Eyebright

Latin name   Euphrasia officinalis
Origin   Europe
Part used   Leaf
Dose   1 teaspoon per cup
                   Tncture 4ml, 1-3 times daily
Constituents   Glycosides (including aucubin), phenols,
                   sterols, choline, volatile oil, tannins
Primary actions Anti-inflammatory
                   Astringent

Secondary actions   Antibacterial
How it works   Tannins coagulate bacterial protein, so
                      provide relief from catarrhal infection on
                      direct application to eyes and throat. Phenols
                      are also antibacterial. The whole herbal
                      extract is astringent, that is it checks
                      secretions, especially that of mucus but the
                      exact compounds responsible have not been
                      identified. It is possible that aucubin – a
                      glycoside – and the saponins are responsible
                      as these are present in several other 'chest
                      herbs'.
Growing guide   Eyebright is thought to be dependent on
                      grass, so is best cultivated in meadow-type
                      planting.

Liquorice

Latin name   Glycyrrhiza glabra
Origin   Europe, Asia
Part used   Rhizome
Dose   1 teaspoon per cup
                      Tincture 4ml, 1-3 times daily
Constituents   Glycosides, saponins, flavonoids, bitters,
                      volatile oil, coumarins, polysaccharides,
                      sterols
Primary action   Anti-inflammatory
Secondary actions   Expectorant
                      Emollient
How it works   The glycosides produce an effect on the
                      adrenal gland to make the body adapt to

inflammation better, growing and repairing tissue. It produces (via the polysaccharides) a soothing lining in the stomach, which appears to have a reflex action in calming coughs. A traditional remedy for coughs was to boil liquorice, linseed, raisins and lemon for a linctus. Its volatile oil and coumarins are anti-spasmodic. Most of the actions mentioned so far are better known for their action in the stomach and digestive tract, so their effect on the respiratory system is thought to be via reflex from there. It also contains saponins which are noted for their expectorant action, thinning mucus and normalising secretions from cells.

Growing guide   Used to be grown in Britain, in warm, sandy soil. Could be tried if fresh rhizomes are available.

Caution   Although the whole root extract is thought to have a balanced action, glycirrhizin is known, on its own, to raise blood pressure. People with very high blood pressure should avoid taking liquorice, and those with moderately raised pressure should not exceed doses advised.

ANTIBACTERIALS

Eucalyptus	Pine	Thyme
Garlic	Sage	

Eucalyptus

Latin name	Eucalyptus globulus
Origin	Australia
Part used	Leaf
Dose	1 teaspoon per cup, 1-3 times daily generally used as an inhalant, using essential oil, but can be drunk as a tea.
Constituents	Volatile oil (including pinene, camphor), phenols, flavonoids
Primary actions	Antibacterial
	Decongestant
How it works	The phenols and volatile oil combine to give a strong antibacterial effect as well as irritating the mucus membrane. This produces thin, free-flowing mucus, which relieves nasal and bronchial congestion. It can be drunk as a tea where the flavonoids are anti-inlammatory because they stabilise the blood vessel walls and help reduce swelling.
Growing guide	Eucalyptus can be grown in Britain but is a large tree and the oil yield is low. Pot-grown trees can be kept small and provide fragrant tea as well as pot-pourri.

Garlic

Latin name	Allium sativa
Origin	World-wide
Part used	Bulb
Dose	1 clove, crushed, 3 times daily for 2-3 days (acute), 1 clove daily for long-term use
Constituents	Volatile oil, mucilage, sulphur compounds, flavonoids
Primary actions	Antibacterial
	Circulatory tonic
Secondary action	Expectorant
How it works	When garlic is crushed the sulphur compounds are activated by an enzyme which produces a powerful antibacterial compound. This is highly volatile and diffusive – it penetrates tissues in the lungs from the blood stream and is effective against a number of bacteria. Garlic is also well known for its effects in the circulatory system, inhibiting clots, lowering cholesterol and reducing blood pressure.
Growing guide	Plant out individual cloves in late autumn in a warm, sunny spot.

Pine

Latin name	Pinus sylvestris
Origin	Europe, America
Part used	Essential oil from leaves and wood
Dose	2-3 drops of essential oil in 100ml of steaming water, inhaled

Constituents	Volatile oil (including pinene, camphor, caryophilline, chamazulene)
Primary action	Antibacterial
Secondary actions	Expectorant
	Decongestant
How it works	The volatile oil is extremely complex. Its constituents combine to give it a strong antibacterial effect. Other constituents, such as chamazulenes, are mildly anti-spasmodic, acting by absorption directly into the bronchial muscle. The camphor is decongestant by irritating mucous membranes, which then produce thinner, free flowing secretions.
Growing guide	Only suitable for very large gardens.

Sage

Latin name	Salvia officinalis
Origin	Europe
Part used	Leaf
Dose	1 teaspoon per cup
	Tincture 4ml, 1-3 times daily
Constituents	Volatile oil, bitters, tannins, flavonoids, oestrogenic compounds, phenols (including rosemarinic acid), saponins
Primary actions	Antibacterial
	Hormonal agent
Secondary actions	Digestive tonic
How it works	The complex volatile oil is mainly antibacterial, supported by closely associated

phenols. These are diffusive, that is they can penetrate tissues, including the brain, from the blood stream. Tannins are directly antibacterial, by coagulating infectious proteins. They act in the mouth and throat, which has given sage its long reputation as a gargle for sore throats. Bitter compounds stimulate the flow of digestive juices, so have a tonic action.

Thyme

(see Expectorants)

ANTI-SPASMODICS or ANTI-TUSSIVES

Angelica	Cramp bark
Aniseed	Wild cherry bark

Angelica

Latin name	Angelica sinensis
Origin	Europe
Part used	Root
Dose	¹/₂ teaspoon per cup
	Tincture 2ml, 1-3 times daily
Constituents	Volatile oil (including caryophyllene, pinene), coumarins, flavonoids
Primary actions	Anti-spasmodic
	Expectorant
Secondary actions	Antibacterial
	Tonic

How it works The volatile oil is mildly antibacterial, which diffuses into the lungs and through the bronchial tree. Coumarins are anti-spasmodic, acting on muscles in the digestive and respiratory system. Flavonoids help to prevent blood vessels from leaking which reduces inflammatory swelling. Angelica has a long history as a chest and digestive tonic although it isn't noticeably bitter.

Growing guide Grow as an annual from seed under glass in spring, will tolerate some shade. Can reach 6ft!

Caution Regular use can increase skin photo-sensitivity.

Aniseed

Latin name Pimpinella anisum

Origin Asia, Africa

Part used Seed

Dose $1/2$ teaspoon per cup
Tincture 2ml, 1-3 times daily

Constituents Volatile oil (including pinene, caryophyllene), coumarins, flavonoids, choline

Primary action Anti-spasmodic

Secondary actions Expectorant
Antibacterial

How it works The volatile oil contains antibacterial compounds such as caryophyllene as well as constituents which increase the activity of the

ciliary hairs in the respiratory system.
Coumarins and other elements of the volatile
oil are strongly anti-spasmodic. This action
supports its traditional use in asthma and
bronchitis.

Growing guide   This umbelifer needs more than British
summer to ripen its seed.

Cramp Bark

Latin name	Viburnum opulus
Origin	Europe, America
Part used	Bark
Dose	1 teaspoon per cup
	Tincture 4ml, 1-3 times daily
Constituents	Glycosides, tannins, coumarins, valerianic acid, salicoside, bitters
Primary action	Anti-spasmodic
Secondary actions	Sedative
	Tonic
How it works	The coumarins are responsible for its anti-spasmodic action on muscles in bronchi, blood vessels and digestive system. Valerianic acid contributes to the mild sedative action. The bitters increase digestive secretions, so have a general tonic effect. Salicoside is mildly pain-relieving and anti-inflammatory. Arbutin is antibacterial, notably in the urinary system.
Growing guide	This is a very attractive garden bush, also known as snowball tree, as it carries creamy-

green flowers in very early spring.

Wild cherry bark

Latin name	Prunus serotina
Origin	America
Part used	Bark
Dose	1 teaspoon per cup
	Tincture 4ml, 1-3 times daily
Constituents	Cyanogenic glycosides, coumarins, benzoic acid, tannins, bitters
Primary actions	Anti-spasmodic
Secondary actions	Sedative
	Tonic
How it works	The cyanogenic glycosides are mainly responsible for the sedative quality. Coumarins support this with an anti-spasmodic effect on bronchial and digestive muscle. Benzoic acid is mildly anti-bacterial, tannins have this effect where they have direct contact on mouth, throat and digestive tract linings. The bitters stimulate secretion of digestive juices. Wild Cherry Bark is not expectorant, so it is used for dry coughs where no extra mucus is formed. Especially useful to prevent coughing at night, most often taken as a syrup.
Growing guide	Large tree, not suitable for small gardens, no known specimens in Britain.

BRONCHO-DILATORS AND DECONGESTANTS

This group includes **datura** and **ephedra** which are not available over the counter. They work on the same principle as conventional broncho-dilators and decongestants but are milder and have fewer side-effects. You must consult a qualified medical herbalist to obtain these.

IMMUNO-STIMULANTS or ANTI-INFECTIVES

Echinacea	Siberian ginseng

Echinacea

Latin name	Echinacea purpurea
Origin	America
Part used	Root
Dose	1 teaspoon per cup
	Tincture 4ml, 1-3 times daily
Constituents	Polysaccharides, polyacetylenes, volatile oil (including humulene, caryophyllene), alkaloids (including tussilagine), flavonoids, bitters
Primary action	Anti-infective
Secondary action	Anti-tumour
How it works	There is a large amount of modern research into echinacea's action. It appears that the polysaccharides are mainly responsible for making more immune cells, such as interleukins and interferon. Echinacea also appears to make immune cells such as

macrophages more efficient and prevents bacteria from making chemicals which allow them to penetrate human tissue. These effects occur directly on contact and also via the bloodstream. The bitters (including humulene) are mildly tonic and relaxing to digestion.

Growing guide   Grow from seed planted under glass. Easy to grow but protect from slugs.

Caution   Echinacea root causes an intense tingling in the mouth which is temporary and not dangerous. It may last 1-2 minutes and cause increased salivation. Research has not determined whether echinacea is safe for those with auto-immune diseases such as multiple sclerosis and lupus erythematosis.

Siberian ginseng

Latin name   Eleutherococcus senticosus
Origin   Europe
Dose $1/2$ teaspoon per cup
   Tincture 2ml, 1-3 times daily
Constituents   Saponins, glycosides, volatlile oil
Primary action   Tonic
Secondary action   Anti-infective
How it works   Although there is much clinical research into this member of the ginseng family, not much is known as to the exact mechanism of its action. It is observed to increase natural (endogenous) cortisone as well as sexual

hormones, improving resistance to physical stress and fatigue. It was reported to reduce the incidence of respiratory infections in Russian factory workers but the evidence was collected under highly charged political circumstances and may not be reliable.

Growing guide   No information is available on cultivation in Britain, which is possible in theory.

EMOLLIENTS

Linseed	Marshmallow	Slippery elm

Linseed

Latin name	Linum usitatissimum
Origin	Worldwide
Part used	Seed
Dose	2 teaspoons in $1/2$ cup cold water, 1-3 times daily
Constituents	Fixed oil, mucilage, cyanogenic glycosides, pectin
Primary actions	Emollient
	Expectorant
Secondary actions	Laxative
	Healing
How it works	The mucilage and pectin form a temporary protective layer over digestive linings, diminishing stimulation of nerve endings. This action is transferred by reflex to the respiratory linings. Linseed is also rich in

essential fatty acids which form the building blocks of secretory cell linings, maintaining them in perfect condition for their functions. Cyanogenic glycosides contribute an anti-spasmodic effect via the bloodstream. There is a tradition of using linseed as a poultice on the chest, which relies on the theory that soothing messages are sent via the skin to the respiratory linings. It was frequently boiled with liquorice and raisins for a cough medicine. It is best soaked for one or two hours in cold water before using.

Growing guide   Easily grown from seed but really a field crop because of the quantity required.

Marshmallow

Latin name	Althaea officinalis
Origin	Europe
Part used	Root
Dose	1 teaspoon per cup, 1-3 cups daily, cold-soaked for 1-2 hours before using
Constituents	Mucilage, coumarins, tannins, sterols, phenols, flavonoids, salicylic acid, asparagin
Primary actions	Emollient
	Expectorant
Secondary actions	Diuretic
	Antibacterial
How it works	The mucilage forms a temporary protective layer over digestive linings, diminishing stimulation of nerve endings. This action is

transferred by reflex to respiratory linings.
Marshmallow contains phenols and tannins
which are antibacterial by their astringent
and chemical action. Coumarins relax
bronchial and digestive muscle. Flavonoids
stabilise the blood vessel walls, reducing
leaking and swelling.

Growing guide   Easy to grow from seed or, more commonly,
by dividing a plant from a nursery. Tolerates
damp and semi-shade.

Slippery elm

Latin name	Ulmus fulvus
Origin	America
Part used	Inner bark
Dose	1 teaspoon in $1/2$ cup water, 1-3 times daily. To be cold soaked for 1-2 hours before use.
Constituents	Mucilage, tannins
How it works	Slippery elm has a very simple action. The mucilage works like that in linseed and marshmallow. It was often prepared with lemon, sugar and a touch of cayenne (chilli) pepper!
Growing guide	Large tree which has not been grown in Britain.

ANTI-ALLERGENICS

Chamomile	Ephedra

Chamomile

Latin name	Matricaria chamomilla. This plant has undergone more name changes than any other in medicinal use. Check with your supplier for exact identification
Origin	Europe
Part used	Flowers
Dose	1 teaspoon per cup Tincture 4ml, 1-3 times daily
Constituents	Flavonoids, bitters, glycosides, coumarins, polysaccharides, tannins, phenols, salicylates, valerianic acid, volatile oil (including chamazuline)
Primary actions	Relaxant Digestive tonic Anti-spasmodic
Secondary actions	Anti-allergenic Anti-inflammatory
How it works	The volatile oil is anti-inflammatory and pain-relieving, penetrating lungs and the bronchial tree by inhalation and via the bloodstream. Coumarins are strongly anti-spasmodic, acting on digestive and respiratory muscles. The polysaccharides stimulate the immune system to reduce infection but also reduce mucous membrane

reaction to allergens (decreasing mast cells for example). These actions work together to relieve some of the symptoms of asthma and hayfever. Chamomile has many more effects and constituents which are not included here.

Growing guide   Grow from seed sown directly in a warm spot, well-drained soil. Grows well in pots

Ephedra

(see Broncho-dilators and decongestants)

CIRCULATORY TONICS

Chilli	Horseradish
Ginger	Mustard

These were sometimes used in poultices on the chest but more often as an addition to cough medicines. Their irritant chemicals raise blood flow and heat in target organs such as lungs.

Chilli or Cayenne

Latin name   Capsicum minimum
Origin   America
Part used   Fruit
Dose   Depends largely on individual tolerance. Start with one tiny pinch of powder, or one drop of tincture in a little warm water, once or twice daily. Work up to a maximum of 1ml, 1-2 times daily

Constituents	Pungent element (capsaicin), flavonoids, steroidal saponins
Primary actions	Circulatory stimulant
	Digestive tonic
	Pain-reliever
Secondary actions	Anti-spasmodic
	Antiseptic
How it works	The pungent (hot) compound, capsaicin, causes blood vessels to dilate and skin to sweat by irritation. This creates a feeling of warmth and improves blood flow to all parts. It also stimulates digestive secretions from the mouth onwards, so absorption of nutrients is enhanced. Applied to the skin it produces a strong warming effect called rubefacience.
Growing guide	Greenhouse only, or sunny window-ledge, very attractive and great fun!
Caution	Can cause pain on an ulcerated stomach or gullet, and intense heat in the mouth. Traces on fingers can cause irritation if rubbed into eyes, so care must be taken with the dose and with washing hands after massage.

Ginger

Latin name	Zingiber
Origin	Asia
Part used	Rhizome
Dose	1/3 teaspoon to 1 cup, 1-2 cups daily
	Tincture 2ml, daily

Constituents	Volatile oil (camphene), eucalyptine (shogaols), gingerols
Primary actions	Circulatory tonic
	Stimulating digestive tonic
Secondary action	Anti-inflammatory
How it works	The shogaols (produced in drying) act on the stomach wall, reducing sensitivity and nausea. This makes it suitable for delicate digestions. The shogaols also cause dilation of blood vessels, easing flow of blood both to the digestive system and the peripheral areas of the body. They are also known to inhibit prostaglandin synthesis and so reduce inflammation.
Growing guide	Can be grown as an attractive indoor plant but will not produce large rhizomes.

Horseradish

Latin name	Armoracia rusticana
Origin	Europe
Part used	Root
Dose	Usually taken as sauce on nut, meat and fish dishes. Very pungent, so small amounts such as $1/2$ teaspoon taken in a bland base such as cream or yoghurt
Constituents	Glucosilinates (mustard oils), Vitamins B and C, asparagine, bitter resin
Primary actions	Digestive tonic
	Circulatory stimulant
Secondary actions	Diuretic

How it works   When eaten the mustard oils in horseradish
                    stimulate digestive secretions, so enhance
                    absorption of nutrients. They also increase
                    circulation by dilating blood vessels and
                    cause sweating. When applied to the skin the
                    infused oil creates heat (it is rubefacient)
                    which helps to relax muscles below.
                    Asparagine increases the elimination of water
                    via the kidneys. Best taken as a regular part of
                    the diet.

Caution   Like all members of the brassica family it
                    should not be overused, as the glucosilinates
                    reduce thyroid activity in large doses.
                    Horseradish oil may be too hot for sensitive
                    skins. Can cause pain if stomach is ulcerated.

Growing guide   Grown easily outdoors from root cuttings.
                    Will need to be isolated as it spreads easily –
                    some people grow it in dustbins. Warning –
                    roots may go down 4ft or more!

Mustard

Latin name   Brassica nigra
Origin   Europe
Part used   Seed
Dose   1/2 teaspoon, 1-2 times daily, usually taken as
                    sauce with food, also applied as infused oil
                    and in foot-baths (1 dessertspoon to 2 pints
                    water, infused until lukewarm)
Constituents   Glucosilinates (mustard oils), sinapin, fixed
                    oil, mucilage

How it works	The hot mustard oils, taken internally produce irritation, feelings of warmth and sweating, which is accompanied by blood vessel dilation. Applied to the skin it warms, relaxes muscles and increases blood flow through the tissues beneath. Mustard foot baths have been satirised by cartoonists, but are a surprisingly effective way of counteracting mild hypothermia.
Growing guide	Large amounts are needed to obtain enough seed for use, so mustard is more suitable to farm or commercial development

BITTER DIGESTIVE TONICS

Agrimony	Vervein
Gentian	Wormwood

Agrimony

Latin name	Agrimonia eupatoria
Origin	Europe
Part used	Leaf
Dose	1 teaspoon per cup
	Tincture 4ml, 1-3 times daily
Primary actions	Astringent
	Bitter tonic
Secondary action	Anti-viral
Constituents	Volatile oil, tannins, bitters, flavonoids, polysaccharides, coumarins

How it works	Agrimony is mildly bitter, so acts as a liver and digestive tonic. The tannins are responsible for the astringent action on the bowel wall. Coumarins are anti-spasmodic, working directly on smooth muscle. Polysaccharides are immune stimulant, which may account for its reputation as an anti-viral.Flavonoids stabilise capillary membranes, reducing inflammation (this is a long-term action).
Growing guide	Sow directly. Prefers dry sunny soil, will tolerate a position next to a hedge or wall.

Gentian

Latin name	Gentiana lutea
Origin	Europe
Part used	Root
Dose	1/2 teaspoon per cup Tincture 2ml, 1-3 times daily
Constituents	Bitters, glycosides, flavonoids, phenols, alkaloids
Primary action	Bitter tonic
Secondary action	Antibacterial
How it works	The bitter taste is very strong and stimulates the flow of digestive juices. The phenols are antibacterial, so it helps to reduce digestive gas as well. The overall action achieves a better absorption of nutrients and so contributes to better health.
Growing guide	Requires special Alpine conditions.

Vervein

Latin name	Verbena officinalis
Origin	Europe
Part used	Leaf, flower
Dose	1 teaspoon per cup, 1-3 cups per day. Tincture 3ml, 1-3 times daily
Constituents	Glycosides, iridoids, bitters, volatile oil, alkaloids, mucilage
Primary actions	Relaxant Bitter digestive tonic
Secondary actions	Antidepressant Anti viral Febrifuge
How it works	Not all actions are clearly understood. Bitters stimulate liver and digestive secretions, unknown constituents act on the brain to reduce sensitivity to pain and increase feelings of well-being. These constituents are probably found in the volatile oil, which is responsible for the anti-viral effect, acting as a repellant in the tissues of the body. This is known as the 'constitutional effect' which French aromatherapists call the *terrain theory*.
Growing guide	Easy to grow from seed directly sown in the soil. Very invasive.

Wormwood

Latin name	Artemisia absinthum
Origin	Europe
Part used	Leaf

Dose	¹/₂ teaspoon per cup
	Tincture 2ml, 1-3 times daily
Constituents	Volatile oil (includes thujone), bitters, flavonoids, phenols, tannins, coumarins
Primary actions	Bitter tonic
	Anti-parasitic
Secondary actions	Anti-infective
	Carminative
How it works	Wormwood's volatile oil is immensely complex, containing chemicals from many groups of plants such as pine, chamomile, cedar, mint and rosemary. These are strongly anti-infective and act with other compounds specific to wormwood in removing intestinal worms safely and without griping. The same chemicals are antibacterial throughout the digestive system. The phenols and tannins contribute to this effect. Tannins also protect inflamed surfaces and coumarins ensure relaxation of the bowel muscle, acting directly on it. Wormwood is intensely bitter, so increases digestive secretions which improves breakdown and absorption of nutrients.
Growing guide	Easy to grow but rather a weedy looking herb.
Caution	Wormwood is not suitable for long-term frequent use as the thujone content of the volatile oil may accumulate causing nerve damage.

RELAXANTS

Chamomile	Limeflowers	Vervein
Kava-kava	Skullcap	
Lemon balm	Valerian	

Chamomile

(see Anti-allergenics)

Kava-kava

Latin name	Piper methysticum
Origin	South Sea Island
Part used	Root
Dose	1 teaspoon per cup, 1-2 cups per day
	Tincture 3ml, 1-2 times daily
Constituents	Pyrones, piperidine alkaloids, glycosides, mucilage
Primary actions	Relaxant
	Antidepressant
Secondary actions	Anti-spasmodic
	Diuretic
How it works	Not much is known about the actions of kava-kava, though research is increasing as it becomes popular. The pyrones and piperidines act centrally (on the brain) to reduce sensitivity to pain. Applied topically it is rubefacient and numbing. It also has a reputation for relieving fatigue, so in some books it is referred to as a stimulant. It is best to view it like alcohol, relaxing and

stimulating at the same time, with some effects of intoxication at high doses.

Growing guide   It is not possible in the British Isles.

Lemon balm

Latin name   Melissa officinalis
Origin   Europe
Part used   Leaf
Dose   1 teaspoon per cup 1-3 cups per day
Tincture 4ml, 1-3 times daily
Constituents   Volatile oil, flavonoids, phenols, triterpenes, tannins
Primary actions   Relaxant
Digestive tonic
Secondary actions   Anti-viral
Anti-thyroid
How it works   The volatile oil has a central relaxing effect (on the brain) as well as reducing thyroid hormone stimulation of other systems. It also inhibits the growth of viruses such as herpes by giving a sort of repellant protection to the tissues, and possibly penetrating viral coating. The phenols add to this effect and help to dispel bacteria in the gut. Triterpenes are bitter, so stimulate digestive secretions, and tannins astringe the wall of the gut, alleviating diarrhoea.
Growing guide   You will rarely have to resort to seed, nearly everyone has some lemon balm to give away. It seeds itself like mad, tolerates any soil and will grow in pots.

Limeflowers

Latin name	Tilia europaea
Origin	Europe
Part used	Leaf and flower
Dose	1 teaspoon per cup, 1-2 cups per day
	Tincture 4ml, 1-3 times daily
Constituents	Volatile oil, flavonoids, phenols, mucilage, tannins
Primary actions	Relaxant
	Lowers blood pressure
Secondary actions	Increases sweating
	Anti-spasmodic
How it works	The volatile oil reduces the brain's sensitivity to pain messages. Mucilage soothes the stomach and gut wall and flavonoids make blood vessels less fragile. Phenols are antiseptic and diaphoretic (increase sweating), which induces dilation of blood vessels. The overall effect is to calm and lower blood pressure. Limeflowers is a particularly nice tasting tea.
Growing guide	Too large a tree for the average garden, a most magnificent specimen can be seen at Kew Gardens in London

Skullcap

Latin name	Scutellaria laterifolia
Origin	America
Part used	Leaf
Dose	1 teaspoon per cup, 1-2 cups per day

	Tincture 3ml, 1-3 times daily
Constituents	Flavonoids, glycosides, iridoids, volatile oil, tannin
Primary actions	Relaxant
Secondary actions	Anti-spasmodic
	Possibly anti-inflammatory
How it works	Little is known about the active constituents of American skullcap as most research is based on a Chinese variant. We rely on the tradition of use for our knowledge of its actions. The anti-inflammatory effect is present in the Chinese variety and it is very likely that both varieties have the same constituents. American skullcap is noted for its central (brain) calming effect. Flavonoids stabilise blood vessel walls and contribute to its mooted anti-inflammatory effect, as well as mildly increasing the elimination of water via the kidneys. It has a long traditional use for neurological diseases such as epilepsy and motor neurone diseases.
Growing guide	Prefers damp soil. Sow under glass and plant out in early summer in a warm, damp spot (pond-side, bog-garden).

Valerian

Latin name	Valeriana officinalis
Origin	Europe
Part used	Root
Dose	1 teaspoon per cup, one cup per night

	Tincture 2-5ml, nightly
Constituents	Valerianic acid, alkaloids, glycosides, tannins, choline, flavonoids, valepotriates, iridoids
Primary action	Relaxant/sedative
Secondary action	Anti-spasmodic
How it works	Valerianic acid and valepotriates reduce excitability of brain and feelings of anxiety. Best used at night as it is on the borderline between relaxants and sedatives. Flavonoids are mildly diuretic (increase water elimination).
Growing guide	Sow directly in a sunny spot with damp soil in early spring.

Vervein

(see Bitter digestive tonics)

~ 3 ~

Growing and making your own herbal remedies

You can prepare herbs in a wide variety of ways to bring improvements in asthma and bronchitis.

Types of herbal preparation

Oral remedies

Oral remedies are swallowed in measured doses. They include:

- teas
- tinctures
- syrups
- pills.

Topical remedies

Topical remedies are applied to the skin and include:
- creams
- oils
- baths
- plasters and poultices.

Oral remedies

Teas or tisanes

Teas, also called tisanes, can be made directly from dried herbs.

- Leaves and flowers require five minutes steeping in freshly boiled water. Always place a saucer or cover on the cup to keep in valuable aromatic ingredients. This is known as an **infusion**.
- Roots, barks, seeds and berries need boiling for five minutes in a covered pan. This is called a **decoction**.

The usual dose is one rounded teaspoon per cup (about 4g to 165ml). Regular use means one or two cups per day for several weeks. Infusions and decoctions can be drunk cold, and any flavouring can be added after steeping or boiling.

- To make an infusion steep cut leaf or flower for 5-10 minutes in boiling water.
- To make a decoction boil cut root or bark for 5-10 minutes on the stove.

Many people ask if the dosage of dried herbs should be different from fresh herbs. As the loss of chemicals in drying may balance the greater concentration due to loss of water, it is best to simply use the same amounts whether fresh or dry. Some herbs such as lemon calm, chamomile and basil taste better when fresh and are slightly more effective, but most herbs keep their medicinal qualities very well if dried carefully. Roots and barks often improve their taste with drying as they lose their acrid components and become sweeter.

Measurements

1ml = 1g
1 teaspoon = 5ml
1cup = 165ml

Tinctures are usually 1: 5, or one part herb to five parts alcoholic liquid.

Doses for adults

Adults will usually require one to three cups a day of herbal teas (whether infused or decocted), using one teaspoon of herb per cup.

Adult doses of tincture vary according to the herbs used in them. Usually half a teaspoon of single herb tinctures, three times daily, is required. With great care you can get 80 drops onto a 5ml teaspoon, so you can work out your dose that way too, and use the formula given below to calculate a child's dose. The amount of alcohol in one teaspoon of tincture is very small but you can add the remedy to hot water and allow some of the alcohol to evaporate if you wish. Elderly people may require different doses, as body weight falls or if digestion isn't as good. One should start with a lower dose and work up if required.

Doses for children

Children require smaller doses. There are some formulae
which can be used, based on a child's age. For example,
divide the child's age by twenty, to give the proportion of
an adult dose, i.e. 6(years) divided by 20 = 3/10 adult
dose. You also have to take into account the child's body
weight, giving less if a child is underweight for his/her
age.

Common doses for teas are: a tablespoon of tea to a
child under 5, half a cup for a child from 5 to 10 years
and a full cup from 11 years onwards. Beatrice Potter
seems to agree, as Peter Rabbit was given a large spoonful
of chamomile tea after he had over-eaten in Mr
McGregor's garden!

Making your own formula

You can combine herbs in tincture or tea form to obtain a
mixture of effects which will suit your individual needs.
Start by choosing the actions that you want – for example
anti-inflammatory, antibacterial, and look for herbs which
provide them. It is best to include no more than three or
four herbs in one mixture, and with careful selection you
can choose herbs with more than one action to match
your requirements.

If you are using dried or fresh herbs to make teas, you
should choose herbs which require the same sort of
preparation (remember that roots, barks and seeds need
boiling, leaves and flowers need infusing). You will only

need one teaspoon of your mix because herbs act synergistically as you have learnt already.

Tinctures

These have become very popular in Britain, both among herbalists and consumers. They are made by soaking herbal material, finely chopped, in an alcoholic liquid about 70% proof. This could be brandy or vodka. Generally, you use one part herb to five parts liquid, so 100g to 500ml. Chop the herbs as finely as possible and cover with the alcohol. Turn, shake or stir every day for ten days. This is to ensure that every particle of herb is in contact with alcohol, otherwise moulds may develop. After ten days, strain and squeeze out the remaining 'marc' through a clean piece of material. Keep the tincture you have made in a dry bottle with a tight stopper.

This can be used in place of herbal tea. Each teaspoon of tincture generally gives the effect of a small cup of tea. Sometimes herbal constituents are extracted better by alcohol, so it is a useful way of preserving herbs. In the past wines and vinegars were used. Their trace is found in the nursery rhyme Jack and Jill where Old Dame Dob did mend Jack's nob with vinegar and brown paper.

It is obvious that these are much bigger doses than is often suggested on over-the-counter tincture bottles, where the manufacturer is more concerned with keeping the price and profit margin at an attractive level. Tinctures are more expensive than teas, and you should expect to pay between £3 and £5 for a week's supply.

Tincture of lemon balm
100g lemon balm
500ml vodka or brandy

Chop herbs finely, cover with alcohol, shake or stir daily for ten days, strain and bottle.

Herbal syrups

Herbs can be preserved in syrup but they are quite difficult to make as the proportion of sugar to herbal material is crucial. They frequently go mouldy, however carefully you measure. There are two methods, the first is the simplest but only keeps for a few days.

Syrup recipe 1
Place chopped herb and sugar in 1cm layers in a clean, dry jar, finishing with a sugar layer. Leave for one day. You will find a syrup has formed. You can shake the jar gently once a day until all the sugar has turned into syrup. This may take three days but you can use the product immediately.

Syrup recipe 2
Soak 4g of herb, finely chopped, in 56ml water for 12 hours. Strain and squeeze out the herbs. There should be about 45ml liquid. Add 90g sugar, stir over heat until dissolved, boil briefly, strain through a filter paper or cloth. You should have about 100ml syrup. This must be

kept in a well stoppered bottle in a cool, dry, dark cupboard. The dose would usually be 1 teaspoon at a time for children, and a dessertspoon from 11 years onwards.

Pills

These come in two main varieties: pills and capsules. In both cases, powdered herbs are used. Capsules are usually made of gelatine, although vegetarian ones can be obtained. Most are of a standard size, containing about 2g of herb. You can buy herbs ready powdered and fill your own capsules by hand. It's a very sneezy, time consuming business! Tablets are made by pressing powdered herbs into the required shape. You will need to add ingredients to make the dough stick together and the tablets hold their shape. Manufacturers usually use vegetable gums, but quite satisfactory tablets can be made at home using honey and arrowroot as binders. Pills can either be pinched off and rolled between the fingers or tablets cut by hand from dough rolled with a pin.

Buckwheat pills

2 tablespoons buckwheat flour
1 tablespoon arrowroot powder
4 teaspoons runny honey

Knead all ingredients together. Add more honey if required to achieve a malleable paste. Dust board with arrowroot, roll out, cut to shape, dry on paper overnight.

Topical remedies

There are several forms in which herbs can be applied to the outside of your body. This is known as topical application. You need to remember a little about skin to understand how herbs reach their target when used in this way.

The skin

Skin has several layers designed to keep water in (you suffer dehydration quickly if large areas of skin are broken) but allow moisture out when required to cool the body down by evaporation. It is covered with a cornified layer (dead cells) and wax. Blood vessels are very close to the surface, and they dilate when we are hot to allow heat out by convection. They also dilate when we are emotionally stressed, so we flush with anger, embarrassment or affection. These blood vessels can constrict to conserve heat, and sometimes when we are very angry or upset we become paler than our usual colour.

Fat underneath the skin keeps heat in by insulation and protects some areas from pressure (famously the bum!). Muscle is found underneath linings below the fatty layer. If you want to reach muscles, your topical applications must somehow get through the wax, cornified layer, fat and muscle linings first. Oily preparations do penetrate through these layers to some extent.

One way of increasing penetration is to soak the skin in

water for a while. This can be done in the bath, in a steam room, or on small areas with a poultice or plaster. Belladonna plasters for back pain could still be bought in chemist's until a few years ago. Most people have heard of anti-smoking and hormone patches. These use the same principle. Back to Old Dame Dob and her vinegar on brown paper!

Four ways of increasing absorption through the skin:

- bath
- steam
- poultice
- plaster.

Creams

Creams are more complicated to make. It would be easier to choose a favourite bland cream over the counter and add aromatic oils or tinctures as you wish. If you want to try a cream, try the following recipe.

Rosemary cream
8 parts oil
1 part beeswax
a few drops essential oil

Gently heat oil and beeswax together in a bowl, set in a pan of water. When wax has melted, add essential oil and pour into pots immediately.

Greasy ointments like this are generally not considered to

be good for skin conditions such as eczema, where they inhibit healing and trap heat, but they are suitable for applying as muscle and joint rubs. Their advantage over liquid preparations is that they don't drip on the floor. A cream such as the one described above could be used to make a vapour rub.

Massage oils

This option is useful if you want to use herbs from your garden. Simply pick a handful of fresh herbs, chop finely and cover loosely with any oil – almond, olive or even sunflower oil. Place the bowl of oil and herbs in a pan of water and put the lid on. Heat until simmering and leave on the lowest possible heat for 1-2 hours. A slow-pot can give ideal conditions for making infused oils as it maintains a constant, very low simmering temperature. Spices can also be infused in vegetable oils.

There are many essential oils available now which save you the time involved in infusing plants in oil. The easiest way to apply these is in a carrier oil such as olive, almond or coconut. A few drops to a tablespoon will suffice. You can add a dash of chilli or ginger! Massaging increases blood flow to muscles and breaks down the tension in them.

Baths

Essential oils can be added to the bath. Use a teaspoon of unscented bubble bath or a tablespoon of milk to act as a dispersant. Relaxing bath salts are based on the same principle and available commercially, although they don't smell as nice as genuine essential oils. The relaxing effect is limited, but a helpful contribution, especially at night before bed, and there are no side-effects.

Plasters and poultices

These are used to apply steady heat or continued absorption of pain relieving or relaxing constituents to joints or muscles.

Plasters are made by melting one part of beeswax and two parts of vegetable oil, adding tincture or essential oil at the last minute. Soak a suitable sized cloth in the mix and spread out on a tray to cool and firm up. Apply to the body and cover in plastic or cling film (or paper!) and tie on with a bandage or some tight garment. The most common use is application to chest, back, abdomen and forehead. You could add a hot water bottle or hot towel wrap for extra comfort.

Poultices are similar to plasters, but consist of a 1cm thick layer of fresh or macerated herbs applied to the skin and covered with a piece of material. This was the earlier form of a plaster, but can still be immediate and effective.

Steam inhalations

Nowadays it is easy to buy good quality essential oils so it is simple to make a steam inhalant mix using a large china mug. Some chemists sell a special inhaler cup, made of plastic, which fits over the nose and mouth. You can also use the older method of covering the head with a towel and leaning over a bowl of steaming water, but this is very tedious and time-consuming. You can heat your inhalant mix in an aromatherapy oil burner, using a votive candle and adding your oil to water. This gives a gentle decongestant and antibacterial effect in your room.

Dried herbs can be used for steam inhalation but they are not as strong or convenient. To be effective you need to steam twice daily if you are in a 'bad patch' (you have a cold or the environmental pollution or pollen level is high). If you are using a steam inhaler cup, you must allow the water to cool a little before letting a child use it, to avoid scalding if spilt.

Caution You must never leave a naked flame unattended in a room with children and you must remember to place your burner on a heat-proof surface.

Vapour rubs

You can apply decongestant, antibacterial and relaxing herbs to your skin, by adding essential oil to a cream base and rubbing into the chest or under the nose. This is a useful method for children.

Caution You must check that the preparation isn't too strong as most decongestants are also 'rubefacient' – they heat up the skin and may cause a burning sensation. Peppermint is especially noted for this.

Vapour rub recipe
5 drops essential oil in 30mg of (preferably unscented)
cream, stirred well.
Suitable oils:
- peppermint
- eucalyptus
- thyme
- pine
- hyssop.

Choosing herbs

Identifying herbs in the wild

It is important first of all to know that you have the right
plant. Some botanical families include poisonous and
edible plants which look very similar and can only be
distinguished from each other by fine botanical detail,
like hemlock and valerian which have subtle differences in
stem and flower colouring. You could buy a field botany
guide, as identification of plants is a great hobby, but it
would be wiser not to select your remedies from the wild
if you are a complete beginner.

Fortunately many of the most important medicinal
herbs are garden favourites such as thyme, sage, rosemary,
lemon balm and peppermint. Most people recognise them
and they are pretty unmistakeable. Even where there are
different varieties such as the thymes and mints, they have
the same aroma and characteristics. It is better to choose

the original sort for medicinal purposes rather than a variety because it may be a more reliable source of the chemicals that you need for your remedy.

Herb names

There is a system of naming plants which gives each one two Latin names the family name comes first and has a capital letter, the individual name comes second written in lower case. The meaning is reversed in Latin, for example *Thymus vulgaris* means common thyme. This is the one you would use for cough medicine. Other types, such as *Thymus aureus*, (golden thyme) or *Thymus serpillus* (creeping thyme) will do no harm, but they don't have as much aroma – in fact they put most of their energy into looking pretty! The same can be said for the many lovely varieties of achillea – a cottage garden flower related to yarrow (*Achillea officinalis*). The word *officinalis* in a plant's name means it was known to be used medicinally in the seventeenth century or before. You will need to specify both names when you are buying seeds or plants from nurseries. Addresses of reliable firms are given on page 139.

Growing herbs

Many of the herbs mentioned in this book can be grown in British gardens, some can be grown in pots or window ledges. Growing herbs is a very relaxing and rewarding hobby. Although most aromatic herbs originate in the warm Mediterranean countries, they will do fine in a sunny spot in any garden soil, even on London clay. They do prefer well drained (slightly dry) soil, so adding grit and compost will help them along.

If you are growing from seed you will need to start them off in pots first on a window ledge or in a greenhouse. To sow seeds really successfully, you should buy John Innes compost number 1. This contains lots of sand and fine grit, so that water runs through quickly and the seed doesn't sit in its own tiny puddle of water, which causes a fungal growth gardeners call damping off.

When you have a small stem with two leaves, you pull it up gently and plant in a pot with John Innes number 2 compost. This has more soil, so that fine roots can spread and take in water – it also contains a little more nutrient to feed the growing plant. When your plant is about 10 cm tall or has a few branches, it's time to plant it in a sunny spot or container, using John Innes number 3. John Innes is a type of compost, not a brand name, so you can ask for it at any garden nursery.

Planting out

Locate your herbs in the south west corner of your garden if possible. Herbs don't need feeding or watering once they have extended their roots into the garden soil (after about a week) but containers will need to be watered as they dry out continually. You can even grow herbs in hanging baskets. You can use multi-purpose compost, but you run a much greater risk of damping-off and losing seed before they even grow, which can mean a whole growing year lost. If your plants don't succeed in one spot in your garden, move them! Just dig up enough soil around the plant to ensure minimum root disturbance and put them in somewhere else. Experiment to see what works. There are plenty of herbs to choose from, so find one that suits your garden or space.

- choose a sunny spot
- add grit to improve drainage
- start tender plants under glass
- water pots and baskets daily
- move plants if they aren't happy.

Choosing the right part of the plant

It is important to know which part of the plant you need if you are going to make your own herbal remedies. Flowers, leaves, roots, bark and berries are commonly used but sometimes one part of a plant is edible whereas another part is poisonous. We eat the tuberous root of the potato but avoid the berries and we eat rhubarb stems but not the leaves. Comfrey root stores too many alkaloids which can damage the liver, whereas they are barely present in the leaf. It is common to find stems in with leaves in herbs sold over the counter, as it is difficult to separate them when preparing herbs on a large scale. If

you are preparing your own you should take the trouble
to rub the leaves off the stems as your remedy will be
stronger without this inert woody matter.

Harvesting herbs

Choosing the right time to harvest is also important.

- It helps you to get the best quality of herbs in terms of
  the chemical constituents.
- Leaves are picked just before flowers develop.
- Flowers are picked as they come out.
- Berries are picked as they become fully ripe, while they
  are still smooth and shiny.
- Bark and stem is stripped in the late spring from new
  branches.
- Roots are dug up in early autumn before the first frosts.
  Pick on a dry day, and scrub roots immediately after
  digging.

Storing herbs

Most plants can be used fresh, but it is more convenient
to dry them for use all the year round. The rule for drying
herbs is:

- as cool, fast, dark and dry as possible, with as much air
  circulating around the individual herbs as can be
  allowed.

The best way for home preservation is to hang up small bunches of herbs, loosely tied, in a dark room or shed. A washing-line strung across the attic is ideal. Hanging up in the kitchen will cause most of the colour and aroma to be lost before they dry.

Large roots should be chopped before drying, as they will prove too tough for the knife otherwise. They can be spread out in a single layer on newspapers. The newspapers should be changed when they feel very damp.

Herbal material is ready to store when it is cracking dry. This is a matter of experience. Usually leaves will simply not leave their stems until they are thoroughly dry. Roots should snap briskly or fail to bend under pressure. Berries usually give a little under thumb pressure. They are slow to dry – moulds develop if there is too much moisture so gentle heat (airing cupboard level) is helpful.

When thoroughly dry herbs should be stored in cool, dark, dry, airless conditions because sunlight destroys colour, air removes flavour and water causes moulds. Tin boxes are ideal, however plastic tubs and glass jars are OK provided they are kept in a cupboard.

- Hang leaves on branches upside down.
- Spread roots out in a single layer.
- Dry as fast as possible in a cool, dark, airy place.
- Ready when cracking dry.
- Keep in cool, dark, dry, airless conditions.

~6~

Using nutrition for
a healthy respiratory system

Achieving a balanced diet

People with asthma or bronchitis may have poor diets.
That doesn't mean that diet can cause or cure asthma or
bronchitis, but there are many ways in which you can
improve your resistance to chest infection. The main aim
of a healthy diet is to satisfy the need for energy, growth,
repair and elimination.

Therapeutic diets

A therapeutic diet is one that addresses the needs of
people with a particular complaint, for example, gluten
free diets for coeliac disease, sugar-free diets for diabetes
and so on.

People who suffer from asthma or bronchitis should
aim at a general healthy diet with special attention to the
following:

- High vitamin and mineral content for immune
  defences.
- Decreased saturated fats and increased essential fats for
  healthy mucous membranes.

Daily nutritional requirements

In Britain research into food was started during World War II and was continued by the Ministry of Agriculture and Fisheries with help from the Medical Research Council. They produced guidelines on what people need to eat to keep them healthy and prevent deficiencies. These are called the **minimum daily requirements** and they cover the main nutrients needed by the human body. In America USDA (the United States Department of Agriculture) funds a similar programme, and its books are widely used in Britain.

Nutrition for general health

It is a mistake to look at single nutrients as being a cure for specific conditions, as almost all body processes require a broad range of nutrients to keep them running smoothly. Several vitamins are required to enable absorption and use of minerals such as calcium, zinc and iron, so taking single nutrient supplements is often a waste of time and may in fact upset the balance of some minerals, which may displace others or hasten their elimination from the body.

All human cells need sugar as a fuel to perform their vital functions. Muscles use sugar for fuel as well as calcium and potassium to contract and relax. Salt (sodium) plays an essential role in getting calcium into muscle fibre cells and potassium is vital to maintain the correct amount of salt in the body. All these processes are dependent on each other and on a balanced state of nutrients in the body. This is the state of health which the herbalist tries to restore with herbal medicines and wholistic dietary advice. It is usual to divide food up into seven different categories and we should aim to eat something in each category every day.

You could use these categories to design a food diary or plan your eating for a week.

- **Protein** – cheese, meat, beans, nuts, fish
- **Starch** – bread, potatoes, pasta, roots, rice, grains
- **Vitamin A** – green, orange and yellow vegetables
- **Vitamin B** – meat, wholegrains
- **Vitamin C** – fresh fruit and green vegetables
- **Vitamin D** – fish oil and sunlight
- **Vitamin E** – wholegrains and seeds
- **Vitamin P** – also known as bioflavonoids – fresh fruit and vegetables
- **Minerals** – calcium, potassium, sodium, magnesium, zinc, phosphorus, found in vegetable and animal foods
- **Trace elements** – cobalt, copper etc, found in vegetable and animal foods
- **Fibre** – indigestible parts of vegetables and grains
- **Fat** – butter, cooking oil, margarine.

Daily requirements for nutrients

These vary according to age and occupation (whether you have an active or sedentary job). Here we have taken the figures for sedentary workers. You can use these tables to understand information given on labelling of supplements

- 1mg = one thousandth of 1g, 1µg = 1 millionth of 1g

	Men 35-64	Women 18-54
kcals	2,400	2,150
protein	60g	54g
calcium	500mg	500mg
iron	10mg	12mg
vitamin A	750µg	750µg
thiamin (vitamin B_1)	1mg	.8mg
riboflavin (vitamin B_2)	1.6mg	1.3mg
niacin (vitamin B)	18mg	15mg
vitamin C	30mg	30mg
vitamin D	10µg if no sunlight available	10µg if no sunlight available

Women's needs vary to a greater extent than men's because of changes taking place during pregnancy, breastfeeding, the monthly menstrual cycle and menopause. British guidelines suggest that women over 55 take fewer calories (1,900kcals) and less iron (10mg) daily. The lower iron intake is suggested because there will be no monthly losses due to menstruation and the smaller calorie intake reflects metabolic changes after the menopause.

American researchers give us figures for some of the other vital nutrients which apply to both men and women.

vitamin K	70-140µg
biotin (vitamin B)	100-200µg
pantothenin (vitamin B)	4-7mg
potassium	1,875-562 mg
phosphorus	700-800mg
sodium	1,100-3,300
chloride	1,700-5,100

Canadian guidelines complete the picture, with daily requirements for men and women between 25 and 49 and recommendations for the over 50s (blank means no change).

	Men	(over 50)	Women	(over 50)
vitamin E	9mg	7mg	6mg	
folacin (vitamin B)	220µg		175µg	190µg
pyridoxine (vitamin B_{12})	2µg		2µg	
magnesium	250mg		200mg	210mg
calcium	800mg		700mg	800mg
iodine	160µg		160µg	
zinc	9mg		8mg	

It is interesting to note that Canadian researchers think we need a lot more daily calcium than their British counterparts. This is because they recommend a much higher protein intake which causes greater loss of calcium from the body. You may need to take this into account when you are looking at labels on vitamin and mineral supplements.

Other minerals considered essential for daily nutrition are chromium, selenium, molybdenum, copper, manganese and fluoride. The intakes for these are generally very small figures – from .2 to .5µg. These are called trace elements.

The guidelines presented above are based on the amounts needed to stop you developing deficiency conditions, such as scurvy which develops when you don't get enough vitamin C. Some nutritionists think you need more than these if you have certain diseases, but this is a very undefined area, with lots of claims motivated by the desire to sell products. General health is achieved by eating a balance of all necessary nutrients, which will help the body grow, repair itself and resist infection.

Beneficial nutrients for asthma and bronchitis

Vitamin C

Vitamin C is involved in all energy and repair processes in the body, as well as disease resistance. It is not stored in the body, so you must take some every day. In nature, this vitamin is usually found with a group of chemicals called bioflavonoids (sometimes referred to as Vitamin P).

Vitamin P helps to protect the blood vessels from damage and makes them more elastic. This means they will be more able to withstand changes caused by stress and illness.

Recommended intake of Vitamin C is 30mg in Britain, 60mg in America. British figures are, as explained before, based on the amounts needed to prevent deficiency diseases. American and Canadian figures tend to be higher as they start with a larger quantity of protein in the diet which affects all other nutrient intake.

Vitamin C content of foods	% of daily requirement	
1 cup orange juice	124mg	200%
$^1/_2$ canteloupe melon	113mg	188%
1 cup broccoli cooked	98mg	163%
1 green pepper	95mg	158%
1 orange	70mg	116%
1 cup cauliflower, cooked	69mg	115%
1 cup parsley	54mg	90%
raw cabbage	33mg	55%
baked potato	26mg	43%

You should cut the vegetables just before using and cook them conservatively – that is using just enough water to cover; boil the kettle first and add to vegetables. Boil until just tender, use the water in gravy. This method conserves the vitamin C, which is lost to heat, air and water. Steaming vegetables is even better, but you will need to add salt at the table. Frozen vegetables retain some of their vitamin content, supermarket vegetables may have lost some vitamins in transport. The best vitamin content is obtained by growing your own and picking just before eating.

Essential fatty acids (EFA's)

There are two essential fatty acids, linolenic and linoleic. These are components of fats which are mainly found in plants but found in very small quantities in meat. Wild meat, also known as game, contains far more EFAs than domestic animal meat. They are needed to make cell membranes, especially in surfaces which are constantly being worn away and replaced, such as GIT linings. The human body cannot make these fatty acids and cell membranes cannot be made from any other type of fats. They are part of the group known as polyunsaturated fats, which includes arachidonic acid (made in the body from linoleic acid) and eicosapentoic acid (from fish). This fish oil has beneficial effects on blood circulation but is not used directly to make cell membranes. It is possible that a deficiency in these essential fatty acids (also known as omega 3 and omega 6 acids) may contribute to inflammation of the GIT linings, as they might be unable to secrete protective mucus efficiently.

There are few established recommendations for EFAs. American dietary researchers recommend 6g of EFAs daily, from mixed sources. British authorities suggest between 2-10g daily.

EFA content of foods, g per 100g

	Linoleic	Linolenic
safflower oil	75g	.5g
wholemeal flour	59.4g	4.1g
barley	57.4g	6.1g
potatoes	56.5g	17.2g
green peppers	56.3g	12g
corn oil	50g	1.6g
soya beans	52g	7.4g
sunflower oil	52g	.3g
grouse	31.9g	30.3g
rabbit	20.9g	9.9g
chicken	13.5g	.7g
rapeseed oil	15.5g	10.5g

There are no figures available for hemp, evening primrose and borage oils which are reported to have higher linolenic acid levels than other oils, and are much vaunted as dietary supplements for all types of diseases. Rapeseed oil is also known as vegetable oil, it appears low in the list for linoleic acid but has the highest content of linolenic acid of all the common cooking oils. Linolenic acid is also present in useful quantities in green leaves and beans. It appears from the table above that eating a mixed diet with plenty of vegetables, especially beans and greens, will supply an adequate amount of both essential fatty acids without needing supplementation.

To maintain a healthy digestive system it may suffice to

add 5-10ml of vegetable oils as a salad dressing to a green salad and reduce your animal fat consumption by taking low fat milk, game or white meat (or no meat), reducing cheese consumption and choosing 'white' cheeses such as Wensleydale, Caerphilly, Stilton, Lancashire, Cheshire and goats cheeses as these contain a lot less fat than other varieties.

How to increase EFAs in your diet without increasing calories

- eat salad every day with dressing (lemon and oil)
- eat potatoes and roots instead of pasta
- cook with vegetable oils, use gentle heat for frying
- use soft vegetable margarine instead of butter
- make cakes with vegetable oils instead of hard margarine
- eat beans in salads and soups and add to meat dishes
- eat five portions of vegetables and fruit daily.

In addition, dieticians from the American Heart Association recommend that fat should only represent 30% of your calorie intake. Several books show elaborate schemes of 'calorie exchange' which are quite difficult to follow. By weight fat gives far more calories than starch, so a simpler approach might be to think in terms of a tablespoon (15ml) of fat a day from all sources. This would mean thinking carefully about cakes and pastries, which contain 'hidden fat'. The average pasty contains 50g of fat in the pastry alone! Baking fat is hydrogenated, which converts polyunsaturated fats into saturated fats. These cannot be used for cell membrane building, and leave you no room for further fat intake from healthier sources.

Foods to avoid

Many complementary practitioners routinely ask patients with respiratory problems to give up milk and wheat. This is based on the reported benefits of making this change. Although it is true that some people have problems with milk and wheat protein, there isn't any reliable clinical research to show that consuming either milk or wheat produce broncho-spasm or increased mucus production. Some researchers think that small holes develop in the gut lining, which allow these commonly consumed proteins through into the bloodstream intact, where they evoke an allergic inflammatory reaction in tissues elsewhere in the body. In fact all sorts of whole proteins might 'leak through' by this principle, so that one or two foods could not be identified as the source of a problem.

Dairy foods

Many patients report less catarrh when they eliminate dairy foods and empirical evidence seems to support this. As mentioned before, when saturated fats predominate there may be also a lack of essential fatty acids, which might lead to defective mucous membranes, or even a leaky gut lining, so that there may be some link after all. Perhaps it is, once again, a question of balance. Plant and fish oils should form the major part of the fat content of our diet, with animal fats, including dairy sources, reduced to a minor role.

7

Case histories

The patients whose cases are outlined in the case studies were prescribed tinctures, which were prepared from one part herb to five parts alcohol. Generally equal amounts of each herbal component were used. Tincture was taken in a 5ml teaspoonful's dose, three times daily, usually before meals.

Case 1 Bronchitic asthma after colds

Daniel was an 8 year old schoolboy, living in the centre of London, who suffered regularly from severe coughs, usually lasting a month or so after a cold. When his coughs subsided he continued to wheeze. He had made several emergency visits to local hospitals for nebulisation and steroid treatment. His coughs and wheezing were worse in cold weather, especially when atmospheric pollution was high. He was born a little prematurely, with a blood incompatibility, and suffered staphylococcal infections in his nose shortly after birth, needing antibiotic drops. At 20 months he had chickenpox and suspected whooping cough, from which time his regular asthmatic episodes had occurred. Daniel's family had recently been through a very stressful period, with dual redundancy; both parents had needed anti-depressants to cope with acute anxiety. Daniel's mother thought that his asthma attacks had increased during this time. He had taken several courses of antibiotics in the course of the previous year and he used a steroid inhaler, having moved on to this from a broncho-dilator, bricanyl.

Our agreed priorities were to reduce the number of infections he was suffering, so that he could eventually decrease his use of steroid inhalers, and return to broncho-dilators. Daniel was also advised to use semi-skimmed milk and avoid cheese, to take a fish oil capsule daily with the juice of an orange and to include a dessertspoon of plant oils in his diet daily, stirred into food or added to salads.

The remedy

- Thyme – antibacterial, anti-inflammatory
- Lobelia – anti spasmodic, expectorant
- Elecampane – anti-inflammatory expectorant
- Horehound – antibacterial, expectorant
- Echinacea – anti-infective.

This was taken in $1/2$ teaspoon doses, three times daily, for six months, during which time he had one severe infection – at the onset of herbal treatment – and one minor one. This was a great improvement on his previous record, as he had not needed antibiotics for the second infection and had not been to hospital since the first.

Daniel continued to take herbal medicine from this time on, but the constituents were varied a little, and he started to reduce his inhaler use at the end of the year. He changed from the steroid back to a broncho-dilator at the end of 18 months, and reduced herbal medicine to winter months only.

Case 2   Allergic asthma and pneumonia

Mrs S was a young mother with two children, 5 and 8 years old, running a small business. She was allergic to animal dander, even sneezing when her son returned home from the child-minder, who had two cats. She said that she had always been a 'chesty child' with frequent colds and sore throats. Two years previously she had suffered a bout of pneumonia in the spring and was currently experiencing night-sweats and a persistent cough which was worrying her. She was permanently tired and had poor circulation, with cold hands and feet. She ate a mainly vegetarian diet, but it was high in cheese and low in other types of protein. Mrs S confessed that she frequently missed lunch, as well as snacking on sweet foods. She had taken several courses of antibiotics for chest infections since her bout of pneumonia. Although the possibility of a TB infection was slight she agreed to arrange an x-ray at the local mobile unit if there was no change before the next consultation.

The priority for Mrs S was to clear any current infection,

increase natural resistance and improve general health, relieving fatigue as far as possible. She was advised to reduce her cheese intake but increase beans, tofu, fish and egg consumption.

The remedy

- Nettle – nutritive tonic
- Echinacea – immune stimulant
- Elecampane – anti-inflammatory, antibacterial
- Horehound – anti-flammatory, anti-spasmodic
- Chilli (2 ml in total week's medicine) – circulatory tonic.

The result was that her cough was completely eliminated, she was no longer sweating at night, but she was still sneezing and her bronchial wheezing could be heard through a stethoscope. The first medicine had been mainly anti-infective, so anti-allergenic herbs were added, but the general tonic effect was maintained.

The second remedy contained:

- Mullein – anti-inflammatory, emollient
- Elderflower – anti-inflammatory, mucous membrane tonic
- Nettle – nutritive tonic
- Ephedra – decongestant, anti-allergenic
- Chilli – (2ml in total) circulatory tonic.

Mrs S continued to take this remedy as well as chamomile tea daily for six months, which reduced her sneezing to all but direct contact with animals. She was then advised to reduce herbal medicine to a third of the dose, and stop after two more months, to see if she could maintain improvement.

Case 3   Chest tonic for elderly pensioner

Mr M, an 80 year-old regular customer, called in for a tonic to 'keep his chest clear' in the winter. He was healthy, but to lower his blood pressure he took tablets which were fairly effective.

The remedy

His mixture, one teaspoon to be taken once a day, consisted of:
- Liquorice – soothing expectorant
- Elecampane – anti-inflammatory, anti-bacterial
- Thyme – antibacterial, anti-spasmodic.

Mr M was very pleased with this. He took the medicine from November to March and said he'd never had such a trouble-free winter! He promised to collect another bottle for the next season.

Case 4   Asthma and poor breathing habits

Michael, aged 7, had suffered from asthma since he was 1 year old. His mother thought that he was worse when he drank milk, which he had stopped one year ago, and better in the summer holidays. His asthma was now less severe than in his early years. His mother also suffered from hayfever and his grandfather had asthma. Michael appeared to have a permanent cold, with nasal congestion and copious, thick mucus. He breathed through his mouth and had a rapid, shallow, irregular breathing pattern, with a juddering heave on intake of breath. He took vitamin tablets, broncho-dilators and a cortisone inhalant twice daily. Michael's mother was keen to reduce the cortisone use, so we decided to replace one of his daily doses with a steam inhalation of eucalyptus and chamomile. His main remedy was designed to maintain bronchial relaxation, reduce the secretion of mucus and protect against infection.

The remedy

- Lobelia – anti-spasmodic expectorant
- Datura – broncho-dilator
- Thyme – antibacterial, anti-spasmodic
- Mullein – emollient, expectorant
- Elderflower – anti-inflammatory, expectorant.

Michael's mother was very keen for him to try yoga breathing exercises, as she had heard about this from his auntie, who went to yoga evening classes. Swimming was another option which Michael was more interested in, but his mother felt that it wasn't appropriate in winter weather.

The result was that Michael managed well with one steroid dose daily and went on to eliminate his steroid inhaler altogether. He continued to need a broncho-dilator but the herbal medicine enabled him to use it less frequently.

Case 5 Allergic asthma and nervous tension

Mrs G was an unemployed office-worker who was living in short-tenancy housing, having moved house several times in the past three years. She shared facilities with some very difficult co-tenants with drug related problems, who had recently acquired two cats. Mrs G had begun to experience chest-tightening and a wheezy dry cough, worse after vacuuming, when lying down and in the morning on waking. She had also noticed that her nose felt blocked and swollen in the morning. Her heart sounds were normal, blood pressure a little low and pulse rate normal but irregular. It was most likely that Mrs G was suffering from allergy to animal dander, exacerbated by nervous tension. She agreed with this but was reluctant to tackle the problem with her co-tenants.

The remedy
- Lobelia – anti-spasmodic expectorant
- Eyebright – anti-inflammatory
- Mullein – emollient, antibacterial
- Liquorice – emollient, anti-inflammatory

- Ephedra – decongestant, anti-inflammatory.

A relaxant tea of elderflower, passionflower and chamomile (also anti-allergenic) was also to be taken twice a day.

This brought great relief from coughing and chest tightness. Even though Mrs G caught a cold, it passed without complication. Her co-tenants had moved out, leaving the cats behind, so she was considering sending them to the local animal shelter, although she confessed to being quite fond of them. She continued to take herbal medicine for several months.

Case 6 Bronchitis and asthma at nursery age

Sunita was a 4 year-old girl attending the local nursery school who had experienced a frightening episode of breathlessness after a cold. Her mother said that she had turned grey, then blue, before being taken to hospital. A few months after this she had another cold and fell into a fit of coughing which was only relieved when she was nebulised in hospital. She was unable to enjoy games of chase in her nursery playground as she become breathless when she ran and was sometimes sick. Sunita suffered frequent colds and had been prescribed antibiotics each time. She took a low dose steroid tablet every day. She had been bottle-fed and now ate a varied diet, with soup, salads and fruit regularly, although school lunches seemed to consist mainly of sausage, pizza, chips and beans with no vegetables or vitamin C.

It seemed that there probably wasn't an allergic base to this asthma, but more likely an inflammatory response to infections. Sunita was prescribed herbs to dilate her bronchi, relieve infections and reduce the inflammatory response in the mucous membranes.

The remedy

Sunita was given two remedies.

Remedy 1 for acute episodes
- Lobelia –anti-spasmodic, expectorant
- Datura – broncho-dilator.

Remedy 2 for long-term treatment of infections and inflammatory response.
- Elderflower – anti-inflammatory, expectorant
- Peppermint – decongestant, anti-spasmodic
- Liquorice – emollient, expectorant, anti-inflammatory
- Thyme – antibacterial, anti-spasmodic
- Echinacea – immune stimulant.

This approach worked very well. On her next visit a month later Sunita had suffered no more asthma crises but still wheezed at the end of playing chase. She still coughed in the morning but expelled looser phlegm, and she coughed initially on going to bed at night but wasn't woken by coughing as before. Her mother was very pleased that she had gained a little weight (partly due to the bitter tonic effect of the herbs, and also because of the reduction in thick phlegm). Sunita took remedy 2 throughout the year, which allowed her to continue on the lowest dose of steroid which she hoped to cease in the following spring. She took remedy 1 to sports day and joined in with no problems except a little wheeziness.

Sources and resources

Nutrition – further reading

MAFF Manual of Nutrition (HMSO). A brief guide to the contents of major foods and dietary guidelines with daily requirements. This book was used by every home economics student and teacher from the 1950s until the 1980s when cookery and nutrition became design and labelling!

Identifying herbs – further reading

The Concise British Flora, W. Keble-Martin (Ebury Press). The author was a vicar who spent all his spare time painting wild flowers. This is a remarkable book which captures the essence of each flower and plant. Better than photos for identifying difficult to recognise subjects. Not easy to use, as the plants are arranged in families, but worth persevering.

Exercise

The British Wheel of Yoga, 25 Jermyn St, Sleaford, Lincolnshire NG34 7RU. Tel: (01529) 303233. The main association for yoga teachers and those interested in yoga. Hatha yoga is the type which has most general application – it is yoga for health. This is mainly what you will find being taught in evening classes and lunchtime sessions. It consists of a series of tone and stretch exercises which have been developed over thousands of years in India.

Most teachers include some exercises from other strands of yoga as these are more directly designed to relax the mind and are associated with meditation. Some people with strong religious faiths are afraid that yoga involves taking up a mystic religion. This isn't true – the meditations are designed to make you aware of your mind and enable you to empty it. They can be performed by members of any religious group.

Seeds

King's Seeds, Monk's Farm, Coggeshall Road, Kelvedon, Essex CO5 9PG. Tel: (01376) 572456. Previously Suffolk Herbs, this is the only company in Britain selling a wide variety of wild flower and herb seeds.

Samuel Dobie and Son, Long Rd, Paignton, Devon TQ4 7SX. Tel: (01803) 696444. Dobie's Seeds sell a wide range of flower and vegetable seeds, with a good selection of culinary herbs.

Seeing herbs

The Chelsea Physic Garden, Royal Hospital Walk (entrance in Cheyne Walk), London. Tel: (0207) 352 5646. (Sloane Square tube.) Probably the best collection in Britain, begun in the seventeenth century, brilliant teas and cakes, exquisite pleasure to walk round. Open Sundays from 2pm and some weekdays. Run by volunteers (who make the cakes!).

Buying dried herbs and preparations

Alban Mills Herbs, 38 Sandridge Rd, St Albans AL1 4AS.
Tel: (01727) 858243. *www.lsgmills@care4free.net*
A very large range of medicinal and culinary herbs and
spices, creams, oils, syrups, tablets, toiletries and essential
oils. Small amounts no problem.

Gardening

The Henry Doubleday Research Association, Ryton
Gardens, Ryton in Dunsmore, Near Coventry. The
Association has it's own seed catalogue, run by Chase
Organics, and a magazine for subscribers which gives
advice on organic gardening and news of organic projects
in Britain and abroad.

Gardener's Question Time, 2pm, Sunday Radio 4, repeated
in the day-time during the week, has been offering
gardening advice from a panel of experts to live audiences
for generations. *Gardener's World* is at 8.30, Friday BBC2.

Consulting herbalists

The National Institute of Medical Herbalists (NIMH) 56
Longbrook St, Exeter, Devon EX4 6AH. Tel: (01392)
426022. *www.btinternet.com/~nimh/* Established in 1864 to
promote training and standards in herbal medicine. It is
the oldest body of professional herbalists in the world.
Members train for four years to a Bsc in Herbal Medicine,
which involves herbal pharmacology, medical sciences

and pharmacognosy (the science of recognising herbal compounds and materials).

Representatives of the NIMH sit on government committees and are involved in decisions on the safety of herbal medicines in Britain and Europe.

Counselling and talking therapies

Self-help books are abundant. You will need to read more than one to get an idea of the different sorts of talking therapies.

Patient support groups

These are extremely useful for sharing problems and solutions. Ask in your local library for the *Directory of Associations* which contains all national associations and is updated annually.

List of herbs within their applications

Expectorants

Benzoin
Cowslips
Elderflower
Elecampane
Horehound
Hyssop
Mullein
Thyme

Anti-inflammatories

Coltsfoot
Comfrey
Eyebright
Liquorice

Antibacterials

Eucalyptus
Garlic
Pine
Sage
Thyme

Anti-spasmodics or anti-tussives

Angelica
Aniseed
Cramp bark

Wild cherry bark

Immuno-stimulants

Echinacea
Siberian ginseng

Emollients

Linseed
Marshmallow
Slippery elm

Anti-allergenics

Chamomile
Ephedra

Circulatory tonics

Chilli
Ginger
Horseradish
Mustard

Bitter digestive tonics

Agrimony
Gentian
Vervein
Wormwood

Relaxants

Kava-kava
Lemon balm
Limeflowers
Skullcap
Valerian
Vervein

General Index